# Medical Ethics

# American University Studies

Series VII
Theology and Religion

Vol. 45

PETER LANG
New York • Bern • Frankfurt am Main • Paris

Robert L. Barry, O.P.

# Medical Ethics

## Essays on Abortion and Euthanasia

ACADIA UNIVERSITY LIBRARY
WOLFVILLE, N.S., CANADA

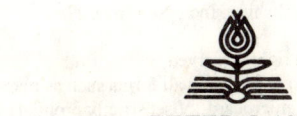

PETER LANG
New York • Bern • Frankfurt am Main • Paris

**Library of Congress Cataloging-in-Publication Data**

Barry, Robert Laurence.
   Medical Ethics.
   (American university studies. Series VII, Theology and religion ; vol. 45)
   Includes bibliographical references.
   1. Medical ethics.  2. Abortion—Moral and ethical aspects.  3. Euthanasia—Moral and ethical aspects.
I. Title.  II. Series.
T726.B29         1989         174'.2         88-36395
ISBN 0-8204-0925-1
ISSN 0740-0446


**CIP-Titelaufnahme der Deutschen Bibliothek**

**Barry, Robert L.:**
Medical ethics : essays on abortion and euthanasia / Robert L. Barry. —New York; Bern; Frankfurt am Main; Paris: Lang, 1989.
   (American University Studies: Ser. 7,
   Theology and Religion; Vol. 45)
   ISBN 0-8204-0925-1

NE: American University Studies / 07

© Peter Lang Publishing, Inc., New York 1989

All rights reserved.
Reprint or reproduction, even partially, in all forms such as microfilm, xerography, microfiche, microcard, offset strictly prohibited.

Printed by Weihert-Druck GmbH, Darmstadt, West Germany

## PREFACE

In the past twenty years, we have seen a circle of killing begun with the *Roe v. Wade* decision come to full close. With the *Roe V. Wade* decision, America was carried over the waterfalls of death into the valley of abortion, and this resulted in the deaths of more than 23 million unborn children. In recent months, however, the river of death has been crossed, we are now entering into the valley of euthanasia. The aim of this book is to challenge the death-dealing ways of contemporary American medical ethics. It is hoped that some of the thought expressed in this piece will help to at least slow if not stop this destructive slide.

In what follows, I wish investigate some of the critical philosophical, public policy and ethical issues involved in the closing of the circle of death and in America's plunge into the valley of death. The aim of this work is to develop the moral and jurisprudential grounds for a public policy that is more protective of innocent human life than what currently exists. I will first examine philosophical and moral issues related to the killing of the young, and then will study issues involved in the killing of the sick and elderly.

I am indebted to various individuals for their support and help in this work. Special thanks are in order to Adolph Barclift for his talents and extraordinary labors which made publication of this manuscript possible. Thanks must be given to Jane Hoyt of the United Handicapped Federation and Nursing Home Action Group for her keen advice and for sharing the fruits of her experience in nursing home advocacy. Joseph Piccione of the National Family Forum provided much needed guidance and consultation in preparing this work. I also wish to especially thank Mr. Robert Destro of the Columbus School of Law at Catholic University of America and Professor Yale Kamisar of the University of Michigan was of great help and encouragement. Mary Senander of the Human Life Alliance and Rita Marker of the Human Life Center both provided a great deal of vital information and help with material presented here.

I am also indebted to the National Endowment for the Humanities for their fellowship granted me in the 1985-6 academic year. Sections of chapters four and eight were taken from a study done during that time of Catholic moral theological and medical ethical thought on the morality of providing nutrition and fluids.

# TABLE OF CONTENTS
## I

## ABORTION

1. **THE PERSONHOOD AND INDIVIDUALITY OF UNBORN HUMAN LIFE** — 1

   A. THE DISTINGUISHING TRAITS OF MATERIAL INDIVIDUALS. — 2
   B. THE MODES OF IDENTIFICATION — 7
   C. IDENTIFYING ANIMATE, SENSATE MATERIAL INDIVIDUALS — 9
   D. THE NATURE OF THE PERSON — 11
   E. THE IDENTIFIABLE TRAITS AND CHARACTERISTICS OF PERSONHOOD — 14
   F. THE CONDITIONS FOR THE PROPER ASCRIPTION OF PERSONHOOD — 17
   G. THE INDIVIDUALITY OF DEVELOPING HUMAN LIFE — 19
   H. THE PERSONHOOD OF UNBORN HUMAN LIFE — 20
   I. ARGUMENTS AGAINST THE PERSONHOOD OF UNBORN HUMAN LIFE FROM CONCEPTION — 23

2. **THE MORALITY OF ABORTION: FACING THE ARGUMENTS** — 31

   A. THE HUMAN PERSON: A BEING OF MORAL WORTH — 32
   B. GIVING MATERNAL SUPPORT TO THE UNBORN — 39
   C. GOOD AND MINIMALLY DECENT SAMARITANS — 49
   D. THE RIGHT TO LIFE — 58

3. **INFANT CARE REVIEW COMMITTEES: THEIR MORAL RESPONSIBILITIES**    65

    A.    INFANT CARE REVIEW COMMITTEES: THEIR ROLE AND FUNCTIONS
        1. The Educational Function of Infant Care Review Committees    67
        2. Infant Care Review Committees and Case Review    68
        3. Policy and Guideline Formation    70

    B.    INFANT CARE REVIEW COMMITTEES: CONCERNS AND PROBLEMS    71

    C.    THE MORAL RESPONSIBILITIES OF INFANT CARE REVIEW COMMITTEES    75
        1. The Moral Duties of Infant Care Review Committees in Education and Case Review    77
        2. Moral Duties in Policy and Guideline Development    80
        3. Moral Responsibilities of ICRCs in Special Cases    82

## SECTION TWO

## EUTHANASIA

4. **THE BROADENING SCOPE OF EUTHANASIA**    85

    A.    MEDICO-LEGAL DEVELOPMENTS PROMOTING EUTHANASIA    85

        1. The Clarence Herbert Case    86
        2. The Claire Conroy Case    89
        3. The Crista Nursing Home Case    93
        4. The "Loving Arms" Case    94
        5. The Mary Heir Case    95
        6. The Ordeal of Mrs. Sharon Siebert    97

|   |   | 7. The Elizabeth Bouvia Case | 100 |
|---|---|---|---|
|   |   | 8. The Case of Mr. Paul Brophy Case | 102 |
|   |   | 9. In the Matter of Beverly Requena | 105 |
|   |   | 10 The Mildred Rasmussen Case | 107 |
|   |   | 11. The Hector Rodas Case | 109 |
|   |   | 12. The Case of Mrs. Nancy Ellen Jobes | 110 |
|   |   | 13. The AMA Statement on Feeding the Comatose | 117 |
|   | B. | THE DOCTRINES AND AIMS OF THE MERCY KILLING MOVEMENT | 118 |
| 5. | ADVANCE DIRECTIVES AND "AID-IN-DYING": PROBLEMS AND PARADOXES. | | 125 |
|   | A. | ADVANCE DIRECTIVES | 125 |
|   | B. | AID-IN-DYING. | 137 |
|   |   | 1. Euthanasia: The Educational Problem | 138 |
|   |   | 2. Overturning the Common Law Tradition | 139 |
|   |   | 3. "Aid-in-Dying": Health Care Providers Turned Killers | 142 |
|   |   | 4. The Paradoxes of "Aid-in-Dying" | 143 |
| 6. | FEEDING THE COMATOSE AND THE COMMON GOOD IN THE CATHOLIC TRADITION | | 149 |
|   | A. | THOMAS AQUINAS | 151 |
|   | B. | FRANCISCO VITORIA | 153 |
|   | C. | JUAN CARDINAL DE LUGO | 157 |
|   | D. | GERALD KELLY, S.J. | 159 |
|   |   | a. The Usefulness of Assisted Feeding | 159 |
|   |   | b. Assisted Feeding and the Common Good | 164 |
|   | E. | DANIEL CRONIN | 167 |
|   | F. | JOSEPH SULLIVAN | 169 |

|   |   |   |
|---|---|---|
| | G. CHARLES McFADDEN | 171 |
| 7. | CATHOLIC ETHICS AND FEEDING THE COMATOSE | 179 |
| | A. FUNDAMENTAL ARGUMENTS | 182 |
| |    1. Criteria for Withdrawing Treatment | 182 |
| |    2. The Nature of Assisted Feeding | 187 |
| | B. SECONDARY CLAIMS | 194 |
| |    1. Personhood and the Duty to Feed | 194 |
| |    2. Revising the Roman Catholic Medical-Ethical Criteria | 194 |
| |    3. Decision Making for the Incompetent | 197 |
| 8. | BRAIN DEATH, ENSOULMENT AND CARE | 201 |
| | A. DETERMINING WHOLE BRAIN DEATH: PROBLEMS AND PARADOXES | 208 |
| | B. THE CONCEPT OF BRAIN DEATH: PROBLEMS AND PARADOXES. | 217 |
| | C. BRAIN DEATH AND ENSOULMENT. | 220 |
| | D. CARE AND BRAIN DEATH. | 226 |
| 9. | ETHICS AND LAW: THE JURISPRUDENCE OF ASSISTED FEEDING | 235 |
| | A. FEEDING PATIENTS: ETHICAL AND LEGAL OPINIONS | 236 |
| |    1. John Paris, S.J. | 236 |
| |    2. Richard McCormick, S.J. | 238 |
| |    3. John Connery, S.J. | 239 |
| |    4. Thomas O'Donnell, S.J. | 242 |
| |    5. William E. May | 244 |
| |    6. Germain Grisez | 246 |
| |    7. Edward Bayer | 247 |
| |    8. Benedict Ashley, O.P. | 249 |
| |    9. Daniel Callahan | 253 |
| |    10 William Smith | 254 |

| | | | |
|---|---|---|---|
| | B. | NUTRITION AND FLUIDS: ASPECTS OF NORMAL CARE | 256 |
| | | Appendix: FEEDING THE PERMANENTLY UNCONSCIOUS AND OTHER VULNERABLE PERSONS: Statement in Support of the New Jersey Catholic Conference, by William E. May, *et al.* | 263 |
| 10. | | LEGISLATING TO PROTECT MEDICALLY VULNERABLE ADULTS | 273 |
| | A. | JURISPRUDENTIAL PRINCIPLES FOR THE CARE AND TREATMENT OF MEDICALLY VULNERABLE PERSONS. | 273 |
| | B. | PROTECTING MEDICALLY VULNERABLE ADULTS | 281 |
| | 1. | THE FEDERAL ROLE | 281 |
| | 2. | THE ROLE OF THE STATES: MODEL LEGISLATION FOR THE PROTECTION OF MEDICALLY VULNERABLE ADULTS | 284 |
| | | PREVENTION OF ASSISTED SUICIDES ACT | 284 |
| | | THE BASIC NURSING CARE AFFIRMATION ACT | 286 |
| | | THE MEDICALLY VULNERABLE ADULTS PROTECTION ACT: SUGGESTED LEGISLATION | 289 |
| | | INDEX | 303 |

# ACKNOWLEDGMENTS

Chapter One, "The Personhood and Individuality of Unborn Human Life" was adopted from an article entitled "Personhood: The Conditions of Identification and Description" published in *The Linacre Quarterly*, February, 1979, and is reprinted with permission.

Chapter Two, "The Morality of Abortion: Facing the Arguments" was written for this volume.

Chapter Three, "Infant Care Review Committees was prepared for the Horatio Storer Foundation Symposium on Infanticide in 1984 and was previously published under that title in *The Linacre Quarterly* under that title in 1985, and is reprinted with permission.

Chapter Four, "Advanced Patient Directives" and "'Aid in Dying': Problems and Paradoxes" was specially prepared for this volume.

Chapter Five, "The Widening Scope of Mercy Killing" was adapted from an article by the same title published in *The Journal of Family and Culture* in August, 1987 and is reprinted with permission.

Chapter Six, A version of "Assisted Feeding: The Catholic Tradition" was published in *The Thomist* and is reprinted with permission.

Chapter Seven, "Catholic Ethics and Feeding the Comatose" was prepared for this volume.

Chapter Eight, "The Jurisprudence of Assisted Feeding" was prepared for this volume.

Chapter Nine, "Brain Death, Ensoulment and Care" was adapted from an article "Ethics and Brain Death" published in *The New Scholasticism*, in May, 1987 and is reprinted with permission.

Chapter Ten, "Protecting Medically Vulnerable Adults" was taken from my short book by the same title published by the American Life League for distribution to state legislatures.

"Feeding the Comatose and Other Medically Vulnerable Persons" was reprinted by permission of the publisher. *Issues in Law and Medicine*, Vol. 3, No. 3, Winter, 1987. Copyright by the National Legal Center for the Medically Dependent & Disabled, Inc.

# SECTION ONE
# CHAPTER ONE
# THE PERSONHOOD AND INDIVIDUALITY OF UNBORN HUMAN LIFE

The euthanasia movement in America started a decade and half ago when it was decided in the U.S. Supreme Court decision, *Roe V. Wade*, that it was legally permissible to deliberately suppress and destroy the life of innocent unborn human beings because they were considered not to be human persons. The principle that certain human beings could be excluded from the class of persons and then killed was given legal and social acceptance in this decision, and it laid the ground work for the legalization of mercy killing.[1] *Roe v. Wade* argued that it was not able to decide when the conceptus became a human person, and it therefore left the issue undecided.[2] Abortion could aptly be considered as fetal euthanasia, for in an abortion, unborn children are killed because they are judged to be either too inconvenient or to be of such poor value, low quality of life, or poor health that death rather than life would be preferable for them. The practical result of this decision was to declare the unborn human being a nonperson that was to be excluded from the protection of the law. At the conceptual level, it was this decision which opened the circle that began the abortion, infanticide and euthanasia movement we are now witnessing in America.

Much of American society has accepted the notion that personhood is possessed by acquisition of certain psychological traits and characteristics and that it is not a trait of our very human nature. In this chapter, I wish to argue that personhood is not identical to psychological personality and that personhood exists as a fundamental element of our human nature, which is thus possessed by the unborn at the moment of conception.

What I seek to do here is to define the formal conditions under which personhood can be ascribed to the unborn. My aim will not be to demonstrate that it is certain that unborn human life is

---

[1] *Roe v. Wade*, 410 U.S. (113) 1973. This decision laid the legal ground for euthanasia because it held that there were underclasses of human beings in our communities who could be placed wholly in the service of others. This underclass was the first to provided with fewer legal and moral rights than other classes of human beings, and as a result paved the way for euthanasia.

[2] *Roe v. Wade*, 410 U.S. (113) 1973.

What I seek to do here is to define the formal conditions under which personhood can be ascribed to the unborn. My aim will not be to demonstrate that it is certain that unborn human life is personal, but that a presumption in favor of its personhood is not philosophically unfounded. The *formal* conditions under which personhood can be legitimately ascribed to the unborn will be described, not by arguing from more traditional principles of scholastic natural philosophy, but by arguing from the principles of contemporary descriptive metaphysics. Invoking philosophical principles urged by the Oxford philosopher, Peter Strawson, I will attempt to argue that unborn human life can be presumed to be fully personal.

Because human persons are material individuals, I will identify the traits and characteristics that distinguish material individuals. Then it will be necessary to show the various ways in which identification of material individuals occurs. Third, as persons are sensate material individuals, I will show what it is that distinguishes these from purely material individuals. The proper traits of persons will then be discussed. And finally, I will show why personhood can be properly ascribed to unborn human life from conception onwards.

## A
## THE DISTINGUISHING TRAITS OF MATERIAL INDIVIDUALS

In order to identify an unborn baby as a human person, it is first necessary to define the various types of individuation and then show how entities are identified as material individuals. Abstracting from its metaphysical essence, we can define an entity as a unified class of particulars.

The most basic type of entity is the material individual because it possesses the following traits which make it the most readily identifiable:[3]

---

[3] Strawson, Peter. *Individuals: An Essay in Descriptive Metaphysics*. (New York, Anchor Doubleday, 1963) P. 44.

> Now, in the respects just mentioned, material bodies appear to be much better candidates for the status of basic particulars than any

1. tangibility, resistance to touch or existence within the tactile range;[4]
2. the ability to be located specifically within the spatio-temporal matrix;[5]
3. retention of its unity of particulars over time;[6]

we have so far considered. They supply both literally and figuratively, both in the short and in the long term, both widely and narrowly, our physical geography, the features we note on our maps. They include, that is to say a sufficiency of relatively enduring objects (e.g. geographical features, buildings, &c.) maintaining with each other relatively fixed or regularly changing spatial relations. Here "sufficient" and "relative" refer to our human situation and need. When we were considering states, processes, &c., we noted that there was no rich complexity of time taking things which were generally discriminable and similarly related throughout the areas of space we are concerned with. But there is a rich complexity of spacetaking things which are relatively enduring and similarly related throughout the tracts of time we are concerned with.

Material bodies, in a broad sense of the word, secure to us one single common and continuously extendable framework of reference, any constituent can be identifyingly referred to without reference to any particular of any other type.

[4] *Ibid.* P. 29. "We might regard it as a necessary condition of something being a material body, that it should tend to exhibit some felt resistance to touch, or perhaps more generally, that it should possess some qualities of the tactile range."

[5] *Ibid.* P. 10.

For all particulars in space and time, it is not only plausible to claim, it is necessary to admit, that there is just such a system: the system of spatial and temporal relations, in which every particular is uniquely related to every other. The universe might be repetitive in various way. But this fact is no obstacle in principle to supplying descriptions of the kind required. For by demonstrative identification we can determine a common reference point and common axes of spatial direction; and with these at our disposal we have also have the theoretical possibility of a description of every other particular in space and time as uniquely related to our reference point.

[6] *Ibid.* Pp. 46-7. The fact that material bodies endure in time and space makes them reidentifiable.

4. public observability;[7]
   5. the capacity for facile reidentification.[8]

If an individual possesses all of these characteristics and traits, then it is a member of the class of material individuals.[9] Thus, a shaft of light or a volume of gas would be an entity, but it would not necessarily be a material individual because neither of these would possess all of the above mentioned traits.[10] In contrast to these material individuals, it is not possible to differentiate one body of gases from another, or one shaft of light from another because these do not have the distinct inherent logical structures of material individuals.

In what follows, I shall elaborate the meaning and significance of these traits and characteristics.

1. **Tangibility and resistance to touch.** The fundamental trait that distinguishes material individuals from all other kinds of individuals is that they display resistance to touch. Material individuals are not primarily distinguished by their extension in space or by their solidity, but by their resistance to touch. More generally, material individuals possess qualities in the tactile range.

2. **Spatio-temporal identifiabilty.** Material individuals are also distinguished by the fact that they exist in, and can be located in the spatio-temporal matrix. In virtually all conceivable instances, identification of an entity as a material individual is

---

[7] *Ibid.* P. 43.

[8] *Ibid.* P. 46. "These considerations taken together suggest that, if material bodies are basic from the point of view of referential identification, they must also be basic from the point of view of reidentification."

[9] *Ibid.* Pp. 43-46. Strawson goes on at great length to distinguish these material bodies from other things such as flashes or bangs which are things but are not material bodies because they do not display the retention of particulars over time that material bodies do and they are not therefore reidentifiable.

[10] *Ibid.* P. 29. "In practice, not many purely visual occupiers-of-space are to be found: some cases that might be suggested, such as ghosts, are altogether questionable; others, such as shafts of light or volumes of coloured gas, certainly do not satisfy the requirements of richness, endurance and stability."

possible because one can locate and identify it within this matrix. Because they exist in this framework, it is possible to identify them as existing "next to", "above" or "below" other identifiable material individuals.[11] The different particulars proper to material individuals such as shape, color, texture and size of specific material individuals do not inhibit but actually facilitate their identification. The inability to know the specific particulars of a material individual will not always limit the observers ability to locate and identify material individuals uniquely as material individuals, precisely because it is possible in many instances to identify individuals by their place in the spatio-temporal matrix. Even though ignorance of the particulars of a material individual might make identification difficult, it is still possible for one to identify a material individual by simply referring to it as the material body at a given place and in a given time.[12]

3. **Retention of Particulars.** The third unique trait of material individuals is that they have the capacity to retain their particulars such as color, dimension and weight through time. Because of this trait, they can be distinguished from such things as shafts of light or volumes of gases which do not retain the unity of all of their particulars over an extended period of time.[13] If this were not the case, then identification of material individuals by their particulars, and not by their temporal-spatial location, would not be possible.

---

[11] *Ibid*. Pp. 13-14. Every particular either has its place in this system, or is of a kind the member which cannot in general be identified except by reference to particulars of other kinds which have their place in it; and every particular which has its place in the system has a unique place there.

[12] *Ibid*. P. 14. This mode of identification works because the proper particulars of the individual serve as logically individuating particulars which permit what Strawson calls "logically individuating description". This mode of identification is dependent on the presence and identifiability of the particulars. Strawson points out that identification by means of proper particulars may not always be easy because the scene might be blurred or because of difficulties in discriminating the particulars, but nonetheless, in most instances, this mode of identification is quite reliable. P. 7.

[13] *Ibid*. P. 20. "Evidently, we can sometimes referentially identify a member of the spatio-temporal framework by giving, or being given, its position relative to another."

4. **Public Observability.** Material individuals are also unique because they can be observed and identified by public observers, and they are not known merely and simply by private experience. Because of this, material individuals are distinct from such private entities as emotions, concepts, perceptions or volitions.[14] This quality of material individuals means that distinct material individuals can quite literally be seen, heard, smelled and touched by public observers, which cannot be done with other private entities.

5. **Facile Reidentification.** Material individuals can be identified again at a different time and in a different place with great facility because they retain their particulars of color, shape, weight and texture over time and in space. In contrast to material individuals, other entities such as shafts of light or volumes of gases cannot be readily reidentified because their particulars do not perdure through time and space.[15]

Facile reidentification is also possible because the above mentioned particulars identified by observers are inherently related to the material individual itself. Observers are able to not just identify the space and time occupied by a material individual, or the particulars of the individual, but the individuals themselves which are the subjects of the particulars.[16]

Having identified the traits and characteristics proper to material individuals, it is now necessary to explain the modes of identification that are employed to identify a material individual.

---

[14] *Ibid*. P. 29.

[15] *Ibid*. P. 31. "The dependent type is the class of what might be called 'private particulars'--comprising the perhaps overlapping groups of sensations, mental events, and, in one common acceptance of this term, sense-data."

[16] *Ibid*. P. 28. Strawson argues that there is a positive answer to the question:

> First is there a class or category of particulars such that as things are, it would not be possible to make all the identifying references which we do make to particulars of other classes, unless we made identifying references to particulars of that class, whereas it would be possible to make all the identifying references we do make to particulars of that class without making identifying references to particulars of other classes? Also see: P. 4.

## B
## THE MODES OF IDENTIFICATION

There are three separate modes of identification employed to identify material individuals:
1. demonstrative identification;[17]
2. identifiabilty-dependence identification;[18] and
3. locatable-sequential identification.[19]

1. **Demonstrative Identification.** This is the most basic, certain and primitive form of identification and it occurs when an observer notes the unified and inherent particulars of the material individual such as weight, size, shape and texture. In this mode of identification, the observer identifies the individual by identifying the particulars are inherent to and properly possessed by the material individual and not by any other individual.[20] When, for example, a material individual is described as being the "ball with red stripes", the individual is identified because of the inherent unity of the particular identified and the individual. It is possible to identify a material individual through this mode because a material individual's particulars are in fact caused to exist and "owned" by

---

[17] *Ibid*. P. 6. Demonstrative identification occurs when an expression is used in a given setting to "naturally apply to a certain range of particulars which the hearer is able, or a moment before was able, sensibly to discriminate, and to nothing outside that range."

[18] *Ibid*. P. 9-10. Strawson suggests that there are other kinds of identification, such as those where individuals are identified through the stories told by others. Here identification is not immediately demonstrative, but is dependent on a demonstrative identification made by the person relating the account of the affair.

[19] *Ibid*. P.37.

> Suppose that all flashes and bangs that occurred could be ordered in a single temporal series. Then, in principle, every member of the series could be identified without reference to anything that was not a member of the series: it could be identified, say, as the bang that immediately preceded the th flash before the last. Now, on occasion, we can work with the idea of a partial sequence, or series, of a somewhat similar kind. We can work with it, for example, in the case of what I shall call a <u>directly locatable sequence</u>.

[20] *Ibid*. P. 4.

the material individual and cannot exist independently.[21] Particulars such as color, texture and tangibility cannot exist independently, for their existence is caused by the material individual themselves. Material individuals "own" and cause their unity of particulars, and when the unified particulars of a material individual can be publicly observed, it is then possible to identify the individual itself. And the particulars of the material individual serve to distinguish for the observer the material individual which are numerically distinct from other material individuals. The reasons why this material individuality serves to distinguish material entities need not be discussed here, as it is extraneous to the issue at hand.

2. **Identifiability-dependence identification.** In this mode of identification, one identifies a given individual by identifying another individual that refers to the material individual being identified.[22] This mode of identification is employed, for example, when one refers to one individual as "the man who was hit by John's car". In such a mode of identification, the man being identified is distinguished by his relationship to another identifiable material individual. This mode of identification is often as reliable as is the demonstrative mode of identification when a clear identification of the related individual is made.

3. **Locatable-sequential identification.** In this mode, identification does not depend on the identification of either the particulars of the individual or on the relation of the individual to another individual. Rather it depends on the ability of the observer to locate the material individual in a series of other identifiable material individuals. In this mode of identification, for example, a material individual is identified as the "nth" individual in the series "K". In some circumstances, identification of individuals might not be as accurate in this modality as in others because of difficulties in

---

[21] *Ibid.* P. 96. Strawson speaks of particulars of individuals in the context of states of mind of persons, and he criticizes theories of the person such as Wittgenstein's which do not permit states of mind to be "owned" by persons. A similar point can be made about the particulars of material bodies, for we have no experience of color, texture or taste existing without "ownership" of them by a given material individual.

[22] *Ibid.* P. 9. It seems that this mode of identification can also be considered as Strawson's "story-relative" mode of identification.

accurately locating the individual in the series.[23] But when accurate location of the individual in the series is possible, identification is as certain as in the other modes.

These are the most general ways of identifying material individuals in order to identify the unborn human being as a person. But for personhood to be identified, one must identify the individual as an animate, sensate material individual, and in what follows, I will describe the traits that permit identification of material individuals as animate, sensate material individuals.

## C
## IDENTIFYING ANIMATE, SENSATE MATERIAL INDIVIDUALS

Animate, sensate material individuals are distinguished by their possession of the following traits:
1. growth from imminent, intrinsic animate causes.[24]
2. states of consciousness permitting responsive reflexes;[25]
3. perceptual thought;[26] and,
4. temporally existing states of mind.[27]

1. **Growth from imminent sources.** What primarily

---

[23] *Ibid*. P. 37.

> Then, in principle every member of the series could be identified without reference to anything that was not a member of the series: it could be identified, say, as the bang that immediately preceded the th flash before the last. Now, on occasion, we can work with the idea of a partial sequence, or series, of a somewhat similar kind. We can work with it, for example, in the case of what I shall call a directly locatable sequence.

[24] This point is made to distinguish individuals who truly grow by acquiring new potentialities and capabilities. Growth is not conceived of here as mere accumulation of material mass, but of development of capabilities and enhancement of existence.

[25] Adler, Mortimer, *The Difference of Man and the Difference It Makes*, (Chicago: Meridian Press, 1968.) P. 106-7.

[26] *Ibid*. Pp. 125-140.

[27] This point is made to simply differentiate between human persons and angels, beings that are pure immortal disembodied intelligences.

distinguishes animate, sensate material individuals from all other material individuals is that their growth derives not from mere accumulation of material from extrinsic sources. Rather growth, which should be construed in the broadest sense possible, is effected by intrinsic powers and causes. In animate, sensate, material individuals, the causes and sources of growth begin at conception and these causes and powers cease at death. It is true that animate, sensate beings require extrinsic natural resources in order to grow, but they are the indirect causes of their growth, for the primary cause of their growth and development in their intrinsic and inherent structure.

2. **Responsive capabilities.** Animate, sensate material individuals are also distinguished by their capacity to exhibit mental states that are respond to the conditions, circumstances, events and processes of their environment.[28] The range of responsiveness of these individuals depends much on the type of individual in question, but common to all animate sensate material individuals is their ability to initiate responses to their environments in some fashion. In a response, an action is taken whereby an individual adopts one course of action as a result of various external stimuli or causal factors. In some sensate, animate individuals, this response is wholly determined by the other extrinsic factors, but other animate, sensate material individuals manifest the ability to act on a wide range of options when choosing a possible course of action. And it seems that what distinguishes the various kinds of types of animate, sensate material individuals is their range of responsiveness to their environments.

3. **Perceptual thought.** A trait that is found in animate, sensate material individuals is the capacity for perceptual thought. In this form of thought, the individual is able to truly think and form intramental images of objects that are perceptually and immediately evident to the individual.[29] In these individuals it is necessary for the object of thought to be perceptually present to the

---

[28] *Ibid*. P. 131.

[29] *Ibid*. Pp. 115. Adler argues that the perceptual character of animal mentation is seen in the fact animals to not make propositions or name objects as humans do naturally.

individual for the perceptual intramental image to be found.[30] It seems that many of these animate, sensate material individuals can generalize, discriminate visual, tactile, olfactory and aural images, and solve problems by trial and error. But in this form of thought, the individual does not respond to environmental factors and causes by judging, reflecting or reasoning through the use of abstract logical relations and principles.

4. **Temporally existing states of mind.** The mental states of animate, sensate material individuals originate and terminate in time, and this is in contrast to ghosts, angels or other incorporeal beings whose mental states might not necessarily begin and terminate in time. The origination and termination of these states coincides with the generation and death of the material sensate individual and with the operation of their intrinsic causes and powers. A person, however is differentiated from animate, sensate material individuals, and in the following section, the particulars which distinguish persons from other animate, sensate material individuals will be described.

# D
# THE NATURE OF THE PERSON

In a recently published book *Unborn Persons*, James McCartney claims that philosophical arguments supporting Pope John Paul II's moral teachings on the absolute inviolability of unborn human life from conception could not withstand close philosophical scrutiny.[31] According to McCartney, John Paul would hold that the individuality and personhood of the unborn from the moment of conception can be made philosophically acceptable. But McCartney implies that such doctrines are philosophically indefensible. To show that it can legitimately be claimed that the unborn are distinct individuals and persons from conception, I will begin by proposing a more adequate concept of the person.

Personhood is not to be strictly identified with individual

---

[30] *Ibid.*

[31] McCartney, James, J. *Unborn Persons: Pope John Paul II and the Abortion Debate*, (New York: Peter Lang, 1987) P. 139.

consciousness, embodied ego, pure consciousness or *anima*.[32] The concept of "ownership" of these states is important because it permits us to identify a material individual as a person.[33] If we did not have this concept of "ownership" of these various states, it would not be possible to identify any material individual as being a person.

The person is a unique animate, material, sensate individual in that it is a "compound individual" because it causes the existence of both material and personal states of affairs.[34] If the person was not the causal subject of these two kinds of predicates, it would not be possible to identify and reidentify material individuals as persons. The fact that persons are these compound individuals means that human states of mind and consciousness can be identified and reidentified.

In the popular mind, the person is identified as being the concatenation of psychological actions and powers. The concept of the person is more abstract than popular notions of the person, and it possesses greater explanatory power than does the ordinary notion. The popular concept of the person as a unity of psychological states is not adequate because one must ask what it is that causes the psychological states to actually exist. A person is a compound individual which causes the development and operation of human material states and human states of consciousness private human experiences such as dreams, emotions, volitions, perceptions and concepts. The person is the formal, final, material and efficient cause and principle of the development and operation of human material states and human mental states, and is the individual that "owns" them because it causes them.[35]

Personhood is a complex notion because the person is the causal agent of both material and mental states of mind. The

---

[32] Strawson, *op. cit.*, P. 99.

[33] *Ibid*. Pp. 93-100.

[34] *Ibid*. Pp. 108-111.

[35] This definition of the person conjoins Strawson's understanding of the person as a compound individual who is the subject and owner of P- and M-predicates and the classic Thomistic person as the first principle of the body. See: Gerber, Rudolf, "When is the Human Soul Infused?" *Laval Theologique et Philosophique*, Vol. 22, No. 2, P. 244.

person can be aptly defined as the soul of the individual, for the person is the unique material individual who causes both these material and mental states. Because it is the cause and subject of these bodily states and mental states of willing, thinking, emoting it can claim "ownership" of them. And moreover, it is the compound individual that causes not only the morphological development of the individual, but also the development of the states of mind that are specific to the human person.[36]

Personhood implies not merely a passive potentiality to receive human states of mind, but rather an active potentiality to cause the existence and development of human bodily and mental states.[37] The difference between these two kinds of potentiality is that a passive potentiality signifies a power to receive a modification from an extrinsic source. But an active potentiality indicates an intrinsic power to cause causes to exist. An active potentiality does not require any extrinsic power for it to cause a cause to exist. This type of potentiality is a power to cause actions, but only actions that befit a certain nature and which are aimed at a certain finality. An active potentiality actually is determined by the final end of the agent, and the type of action caused by the agent is determined by the final end of the agent.[38] Thus, for human beings the most perfect actions debatably are reason, thinking, reflecting, loving and communicating through speech.

Finally, the person is the animate, sensate material individual which naturally claims personhood for itself and which ascribes it properly to other animate, sensate material individuals.[39] Persons are individuals who are self-and other-ascribers of personhood and who do this with intelligence, discrimination, understanding and insight to other sensate, animate material individuals. This capacity sets them apart from other such entities

---

[36] Strawson does not explicitly articulate this claim, but it derives from the Thomistic principle of the soul as the first cause of the body, its potentialities and operations.

[37] Gerber, *op. cit* P. 244.

[38] *Ibid.* P. 243.

[39] Strawson, *op. cit.* P. 100-107.

as mechanical instruments that might also ascribe personhood.[40]

If this is the nature of the person, it must be asked what the specific traits and characteristics of human persons are that permit an animate, sensate, material individual to be identified as a person.

## E
## THE IDENTIFIABLE TRAITS AND CHARACTERISTICS OF PERSONHOOD

It is possible to identify the unborn human being simply as an animate, sensate material individual, but doing this cannot fully explain all of the innate capacities of unborn human persons. A fuller understanding of the unborn human being raises the possibility of identifying it as a person, but to do this may be quite difficult. If this is to be possible, it would be necessary to define with precision what it is that distinguishes a being as a person. If these individuals are to be described as persons, it will be necessary to specify precisely what it is that distinguishes them as persons.

As mentioned earlier, a person is a compound individual that causes human bodily and mental states. Human material bodily states are in many ways no different than the bodily states of the higher animate, sensate material creatures. But the mental states of persons are notably different, and it is these which essentially distinguish persons. In general the following are the characteristics and traits of human states of mind:
1. conceptual thought;[41]
2. syntactical and propositional speech;[42]
3. intentional expression;[43]
4. non-public observability;[44]

---

[40] Strawson, *op. cit.* Pp. 108-9.

[41] Adler, *op. cit.* Pp. 125-7.

[42] *Ibid.*

[43] See: Anscombe, G.E.M., *Intention*. (New York: Cornell University Press, 1957).

[44] Strawson, *op. cit.* P. 84.

5. non-transferrable character.[45]

   1. **Conceptual thought.** This state of mind is found naturally only in the class of human persons, and it enables persons to think abstractly, judge, reflect, reason about necessary and contingent relations, and consider objects that are not perceptually present to the individual.[46] Conceptual thought is different from perceptual thought because it enables a person to think about objects that are not perceptually present to the individual and to gain insight and understanding into the nature, state and relationships of the object being considered.[47] Because of the innate capacity in the unborn human person for conceptual thought it is possible for the person to provide an intelligent understanding of the object, which is not found in individuals possessing only perceptual thought.

   2. **Syntactical and propositional speech.** This is found only in its natural and complete form in the human person. It includes not only lower forms of speech such as description or questioning, but also higher forms such as argumentation, statements about the past and future, and abstract declarations.[48]

   There is an interdependence and reciprocal relationship between conceptual thought and syntactical and propositional speech such that conceptual thought seems to only be possible where there is a capacity for syntactical and propositional speech and vice-versa.

   Because of the capacity of syntactical and propositional speech, persons are able to express their mental states with far more precision, range, accuracy and depth than can individuals who possess only perceptual thought. Those with only perceptual thought cannot provide an intelligent and rational account of the conditions, circumstances and reasons for their utterances as persons can, which

---

[45] Strawson, Pp. 92-4. The non-transferable character of mental states stems from the fact that they are partly caused by the person's body which cannot be transferred to others. Because one's body is uniquely one's own, the mental states caused by the body are also uniquely private.

[46] Adler, M. *op. cit.* Pp. 137-140.

[47] *Ibid.* P. 137. In addition, see: Geach, Peter, *Mental Acts* (New York, Humanities Press, 1957).

[48] *Ibid.* Pp. 136-9.

suggests a difference between the syntactical and propositional speech of persons and the utterances of other animate, sensate material individuals.

3. **Intentional expression.** Persons are further distinguished from other sensate, animate material individuals by their capacity for intentional expression. The uniqueness of intentional expression in persons is that it is conscious, intelligent and rational. Such forms of personal intentional expression as dance, art, sculpture, music, ritual and myth are the types of expression that are found in persons and not other animate, sensate material individuals.[49] There is no indication that other animate, sensate material individuals have the range of intentional expression that is possessed by persons, and while other animate, sensate material individuals might be able to act intentionally, it is not at all clear that they exhibit the diversity and range of intentional expression of persons. That other animate, sensate material beings do not have understanding and intelligent insight into what they do is seen by the fact that they do not purposively alter their expressive actions to communicate new and differing forms of meaning.

4. **Non-public observability of human mental states.** Human mental states are purely private, and cannot be directly and immediately observed by other public individuals. As is the case with other animate, sensate, material individuals, the states of mind of persons cannot be directly observed by other public observers, and they can be known by other individuals only if their traits, content and characteristics are communicated by the subject of them to other individuals.

5. **Non-transferable character.** As is with the case with the mental states of animate, sensate material individuals, the states of mind of persons are non-transferable.[50] The content of some of the thoughts, emotions, volitions and dreams can be communicated to some others, but the actual states themselves cannot be transferred to other persons or material individuals.

If these are the proper traits and characteristics of persons,

---

[49] *Ibid.* Pp. 135-6.

[50] Strawson, *op. cit.* Pp. 94.

the question when it is appropriate to ascribe personhood to individuals must be answered.

## F
## THE CONDITIONS FOR THE PROPER ASCRIPTION OF PERSONHOOD

It would appear that personhood can be properly and legitimately ascribed to animate, sensate, material individuals under the following conditions.

First, self-ascription of personhood would be proper when one subjectively experiences one's bodily states and one's mental states of willing, emoting, reflecting, analyzing, conceptualizing. It would be legitimate to ascribe personhood to one's self when other states of mind could not be sufficiently explained without ascribing personhood.[51]

Second, when one performs kinds of action that can only be explained as resulting from abstract thought, syntactical and propositional speech and intentional expression, self-ascription of personhood would be proper and appropriate because these sorts of actions can only be caused by a persons.[52] What the material conditions are for making such ascriptions to one's self are not relevant to the issue at hand, for all this study is concerned with are the formal conditions permitting ascription of personhood.

Third, it is also proper to ascribe personhood to other individuals, not when the observer subjectively experiences these states of mind in the same way that was done in the instance mentioned above, but when the actions are observed in another individual that can only be accounted for by ascribing personhood to the individual.[53] Thus, when another sensate material individual

---

[51] *Ibid.* Pp. 86-7, 92.

[52] This would be implied by the principles noted in the previous paragraph. Personhood can be legitimately ascribed to one's self when there are bodily states or states of mind that are only explicable by as ascription of personhood. It would seem to be implied in this principle that the immediate experience of actions flowing from or entailed by uniquely human states would justify ascription of personhood.

[53] Strawson, *op. cit.* P. 100.

performs actions such as ascription of syntactical and propositional speech, abstract thought and intentional expression, it would be justified to ascribe personhood to that individual.

Fourth, it is justified to ascribe personhood to another individual when that individual displays actions indicating the development of states of mind, powers or capabilities of a human person because this development results from the causal action of a person.[54] This is the case because personhood is logically prior to the actualization of these states and causes their development. If one could not ascribe personhood to individuals who cause these states to develop, but only when these states were fully and unequivocally actualized, babies could not be considered as persons because they do not fully and unequivocally manifest human mental states. Ascription of personhood is legitimate not only when human mental states are observed to be fully operative, but also when these states are in the processes of development. It is because of this that newborn babies can be called persons, even though they do not manifest fully operative human mental states.

Finally, ascription of personhood is proper and legitimate to other animate, sensate material individuals when they display the active capability to cause and "own" human states of mind.[55] The ascription of personhood to them is warranted because the ascription of other predicates will not adequately or fully explain the observed states of mind. Personhood is ascribed to an infant, for example, because the child has the active potential of performing actions only possible with the presence of conceptual thought, syntactical and propositional speech and intentional expression. Infants are not called persons because they merely have the passive potential to perform these actions, but because they have the active potential as well.

Given these formal conditions for ascribing personhood to individuals, it can now be determined if unborn human life from the moment of conception onwards can be identified as an individual

---

[54] *Ibid*. P. 95. Ascription of personhood in this circumstance is proper because one can ascribe personhood to one's self because one experiences the development of one's states of mind. And if one can ascribe personhood to another when one observes the development of uniquely human states of mind or bodily states.

[55] *Ibid*. Pp. 96-7.

and personal being.

## G
## THE INDIVIDUALITY OF DEVELOPING HUMAN LIFE

Against the claims that the conceptus is not a materially distinct individual, it should be recalled that it is possible to identify it as a materially and numerically discrete individual by a number of means of identification. The conceptus can be spatially and temporally located. It can be identified through demonstrative identification, locatable-sequential identification and identifiability-dependence identification. The conceptus possesses a unity of enduring particulars in its genetic code that enables public observers to distinguish it from its surrounding material individuals. It is also a being that is capable of facile reidentification, public observability and resistance to touch which mark it as a material individual, and its particulars of color, texture and weight endure over time which also show it to be a material individual.

The genetic code of the conceptus is the enduring particular which marks the conceptus most clearly as a distinct material individual.[56] This genetic code endures through the life of the being, and it patterns and in various ways controls its physiological growth and development of the individual.[57] This code is absolutely unique, and is not to be duplicated. This genetic code is the foundation upon which the neurological structure of the conceptus is built. If the conceptus was not a distinct individual being, its genetic structure would be identical to that of its surrounding cells. While the conceptus and the developing stages of life are dependent on the mother for nourishment and protection, they are distinct from the mother because of the distinctiveness of their genetic codes.

The unborn human being can be identified as an animate, material individual, but as one that is different from all other

---

[56] See: Gerber, *op. cit.*

[57] *Ibid.* Pp. 243-246. Also see: Grisez, Germain. *Abortion: The Myths, The Realities and the Argument*, (New York: Corpus Books, 1966) Pp. 113-14.

members of this class.[58] The unborn human being is different from other animate, sensate material individuals because it manifests the development of uniquely human states of body and of mind. This only becomes immediately evident when these states acquire the active potentiality to operate and publicly display their powers, but their existence can be inferred from their later operations. This is not surprising, however, for the mental states of animate, sensate material individuals also can only be known when they come to manifest their powers and operations. Thus, because the states of mind that come to full development at a later stage in the life of the unborn human being are different from those of other animate, sensate, material individuals, it must be concluded that unborn human beings are different from all other members of this class. Because unborn human beings do not at a later point in time manifest the same mental states that other animate, sensate material beings do, they cannot simply be classified with them in all cases.

Given the material individuality of the conceptus, it must now be asked if it is possible to ascribe personhood to human life at that stage.

## II
## THE PERSONHOOD OF UNBORN HUMAN LIFE

The personhood of unborn human beings is not immediately evident because life at these stages does not manifest the operations that are manifested by other more developed human beings. But the operations displayed by the unborn human being are not unnatural or uncharacteristic of persons who are moving toward full maturity. Despite these difficulties, however, it seems that personhood can be ascribed to the early stages of human life for six reasons.[59]

1. There are severe logical problems involved in not ascribing personhood to the conceptus at the moment of conception.

---

[58] Grisez, *op. cit.* p. 14-15.

[59] The fact that the conceptus does not manifest the operations of other more mature human beings is not a decisive argument against its personhood, because personhood is not identified with the operations of persons. See: Gerber, *op. cit.* Pp. 244-7.

The fundamental one is that a decision not to do this necessitates the conceptus, embryo, blastula, morula or fetus transferring at some point in time from the class or species of animals or sensate material beings into the class of persons. There is neither sufficient scientific nor biological evidence to indicate that this sort of "species-transfer" actually occurs in the human species, or in any of the other mammals.[60] If it is true that at some stage in the development of unborn human life there is a class transfer from the class of the sub-personal to the personal life, it is remarkable that science has not rigorously sought to determine that moment, as that event would be more monumental than the moment of birth. It is remarkable that this moment would not be ritually celebrated for it would seem to be more important than conception. If such a species transfer did in fact occur, it would seem valuable to determine what its causes in physical nature actually were. If the causes of this class transfer could be determined, they could possible be applied to other species, thereby making them persons. If it is true that the conceptus does become personal after being generated into a sub-personal form of existence, it would be necessary to posit a modified "succession of souls" theory to explain how this occurs. It is conceivable that such a change occurs in the lower animals, but there is no evidence that such an event occurs in the higher animals.

2. Personhood can also be authentically ascribed to the early stages of unborn human life because of the nature of the person. We should recall that a human being is a person because it causes and "owns" the development and the operation of human bodily states and human mental states. The developing unborn human being is the material individual which causes and "owns" developing human states of mind to exist, and can therefore be considered to be a "person". Intentional expression, syntactical and propositional speech and abstract thought develop over time, and the material individual which is the causal agent of the development of these human operations is the developing unborn human being. Just as a senile human being is also a person because such an individual is the causal agent of not only the operation but also the decline of the

---

[60] Only the most medieval theories of ontogenesis assert that it involves passing through lower forms of existence to higher forms, while modern views unanimously disclaim any sort of "succession of souls" account of ontogenesis. See: Gerber, *op. cit.* Pp. 245-6.

bodily and mental states of the individual.

3. Personhood can properly be attributed to unborn human beings at conception because the unborn human being possesses the active potentiality to cause the development and operation of human states of mind of conceptual thought, syntactical and propositional speech and intentional expression, and this potentiality is sufficient for the ascription of personhood. The mental states of unborn human beings are emerging into full and complete operation, just as the mental states of the senile and victims of Alzheimer's disease are declining in the functional potential.

4. Personhood can be ascribed to unborn human beings because they "own" the bodily states and states of consciousness which they privately experience developing and coming into the fullness of operation. It is implausible that human states of mind or consciousness have an existence separate from material bodies of persons, even unborn human persons. Unborn human beings cause, subjectively experience and therefore "own" their developing bodily states and developing operations of abstract thought, syntactical and propositional speech and intentional expression that they experience. The states of consciousness of unborn human life are developing toward full actuality and reality, and the sensate material being that owns them in their developing stages is as much a person as is one who "owns" them in the fullness of their power or in their decline.

5. Finally, it is legitimate to ascribe personhood to unborn human beings because they have the active potentiality to ascribe personhood to themselves and to others with intelligence, insight and understanding. This capacity for intelligent ascription of personhood is present as an active potentiality in unborn human life, even though it operates only in the more mature stages of human life. It is not legitimate to deny ascription of personhood to unborn human beings because they have only the active potential to ascribe personhood to self and to others because having this capability is a sufficient condition for being a person.

6. Personhood is legitimately attributable to unborn human beings because of the problem of moral rights involved in denying their personhood. If one holds that unborn human beings are not persons, then one would be logically committed to asserting that they do not have the same natural, civil or moral rights possessed that fully mature persons have. If it is true that the early stages of human life are not persons, but at best on a possible trajectory

toward full human personhood, then one could not require of necessity that they be treated as human persons are treated. If it is true that they are not persons, then there is no logically compelling reason why they should not be treated as are all other animals. And as there is nothing wrong with killing and eating animals, so also there would be nothing wrong with killing unborn human beings, grisly as this might be. A major moral dilemma for those who hold that the unborn are not persons is that they would seem to be logically committed to permitting all of the actions done to the unborn that àre done to sensate animate individuals.

However, there are not sound moral reasons to support the view that unborn human life can be treated as all other animal life is treated. And treating unborn human beings as we treat animals is contrary to civilized moral standards. It is precisely because unborn human beings are of the same species and class as are adult human beings that they are to be given the same protections that are given adults. Adult human beings do not have the same moral scruples about eating animal flesh as they would about eating the flesh of unborn human beings and this is because the unborn are of the same species.

Denying the personhood of the unborn creates the serious problem of undermining the foundations of prohibitions of actions that are nothing but brutality and exploitation of the unborn. Critics of the claims of personhood of the unborn fail to see that they are logically committed to permitting actions to which they themselves would object.

## I
## ARGUMENTS AGAINST THE PERSONHOOD OF UNBORN HUMAN LIFE FROM CONCEPTION

A number of authors argue that personhood cannot be ascribed to the some of the early stages of developing human life, and their arguments should be considered.

Joseph Donceel argues that the person can only develop in proportion to the development of the material substratum of the individual.[61] For him, a person can only come into existence when the material substratum of the person is sufficiently formed and developed to receive the more complex spirit that is the person. Thus, Donceel argues that a person can only exist when the "primitive streak" develops because this is the foundation of the neurological system of the human being.[62]

Along the lines set forth by Donceel, Lawrence Becker has argued that the person could only exist if the physical body had achieved a state of "morphological completeness".[63] When the organism has achieved its basic structure and has attained this morphological completeness, then it would be sufficiently prepared to receive a human soul. And similar to Donceel's and Becker's arguments is that of Albert DiIanni who asserts that the conceptus is a mass of protoplasm and he suggests that in the early stages of gestation, the soul is being formed and is not actually present.[64] For DiIanni, personhood can only be legitimately ascribed to material bodies when their period of formation is complete.

In reality, these anatomical developments are caused by the soul, and these writers confuse the soul with the operations and powers of the soul. The difficulty with Donceel's hypothesis is that it cannot explain the causal agency of the "primitive streak" itself, it cannot explain how the "primitive streak" develops. What is the form of agency that brings the primitive streak into existence? In Donceel's theory, it seems to be an "uncaused cause" that enables the person to begin to exist and operate, but it itself is not caused by any other agent.

Becker fails to see that full development of the body is not necessary for there to be full and complete existence of the soul or person. If anatomical completeness were necessary for ascription of

---

[61] Donceel, S.J., Joseph. "Abortion: Mediate or Immediate Animation" *Continuum*, Spring, 1967, Pp. 167-171.

[62] *Ibid.*

[63] Becker, Lawrence. "Human Being: The Boundaries of the Concept", *Philosophy and Public Affairs*, Vol. 4, No. 4, p. 337.

[64] DiIanni, Albert. "Is the Fetus a Person?" *American Ecclesiastical Review*, Vol. 168, (1974). P. 323.

personhood, it would probably not be possible to confidently ascribe it until after puberty, for only then is the individual anatomically complete. Becker and DiIanni fail to see that it is the person or the soul that causes the development and operation of human bodily and mental powers and states and that their development requires the prior existence of the person or soul. The soul or person does not develop and become actualized along with the development and operation of human bodily and mental states and powers.

A further difficulty with Becker's and DiIanni's theories is that they both require a "class" or "species" transfer from the class or species which existed prior to the development of the anatomical structures to the class of persons. These authors offer no explanation of how or why this "class transfer" takes place. Implicitly, their theories would require a modified and modernized "succession of souls" theory which holds that one sort of soul, being, nature or essence would prevail prior to the emergence of the human person or soul at which time another kind of essence, soul, nature or person would then exist. They implicitly hold for a multiplicity of souls in the human person, and this theory has long been discredited by both science and philosophy.

Arguments must be faced which assert that personhood cannot be ascribed at the earliest stages of human life because hydatidiform moles, twins and chimeras are not persons as they are either not sufficiently developed to cause personal states of mind, or they are not true individuals.[65] It is probably true that hydatidiform moles are not persons but that is probably because their developmental anomalies resulted from the placenta rather than from the embryos, which means that true conception never occurred. But it is not true that the embryo, prior to the point where twinning becomes impossible, is not a human being because twins could very be the product of "non-sexual" form of human reproduction.

---

[65] Twinning does not necessarily constitute an irrefutable argument that one individual conceptus has become two, as in some instances two individuals existed from the outset of the conception process. And when twinning occurs later, it does apparently always occur at the same time. There also seems to be a genetic factor involved in twinning such that not every zygote is capable of splitting. And both hydatidiform moles and "monsters" should be viewed as variations on the normal course of human development, but it is highly unlikely that they can be considered human persons because of their disorganized patterns of growth. See: Grisez, *op. cit.* Pp. 24-30.

Opponents of the personhood of the unborn cite chimeras as counterexamples. But, it is by no means clear that true chimeras are possible within the human species. And even if they are biologically possible, that does not mean that chimeras are not distinct individuals or persons.[66] It is theoretically possible that the primitive cells of the conceptus incorporate genetic materials from other cells, but in so doing they can still retain their individuality and still remain persons because they would still be the cells that cause and "own" developing human bodily and mental states.

A much more sophisticated argument against the personhood of unborn human life is presented by Michael Tooley. Tooley contends that it is only legitimate to ascribe personhood to individuals who have:

1) the desire to continue living;
2) have a concept of the self as a continuing subject of experiences and other mental states; and,
3) believe that the self is a continuing entity.[67]

Tooley's argument is somewhat persuasive because he presents what is our unreflective understanding of the nature of the human person. Tooley asserts that it would be possible to ascribe personhood to some animals who might be able to meet these criteria and thereby ascribe them rights commonly reserved to human beings, and it might also be possible to deny personhood to some human beings who do not meet these criteria.[68] Tooley, like Peter Singer, argues that membership in the human species is not

---

[66] Chimeras, or cell populations derive from more than one fertilized egg, are believed to be produced naturally in small numbers. There is some evidence that some individuals actually do have two genomes present in their bodies, one present in the gonadal area and another in the rest of the body cells. See: McCartney, *op. cit.* Pp. 145-7. What these developmental anomalies suggest, however, is that even when there has been a fusion of embryonic cells, it is still possible for a genetically distinct individual to develop.

[67] Tooley, Michael. "Abortion and Infanticide", in *The Rights and Wrongs of Abortion*, ed. by Marshall Cohen, Thomas Nagel and Thomas Scanlan. (Princeton: Princeton University Press, 1974). P. 59.

[68] *Ibid.* Pp. 52-84.

critical.[69] He argues in behalf of this criterion of personhood in order to permit not only abortion of the unborn, but also infanticide for some severely handicapped newborns. He believes that anencephalic, hydroencephalic and persistently comatose infants are not human persons because they do not meet this criterion, and thus he does not see any moral malice in bringing them to death.[70]

Tooley argues that just as there would be nothing wrong with killing a kitten who was injected with a serum that would make it a full person, so also there would be nothing wrong with killing an unborn human being.[71] This is because both of these are "potential" persons but not real ones. Relying on such science fiction arguments is a very feeble way of defending philosophical principles, yet Tooley fails to see that the kitten is undergoing a species-transfer and the unborn human being is not. He fails to see that the personhood of the kitten is extrinsic to it while the personhood of the unborn human being is intrinsic. Tooley claims that the unborn human being is only a potential person, but he fails to see the difference between active and passive potentiality. If the kitten were a simple animate, sensate material individual there would be nothing immoral in killing it *in some cases*. But if it were a true person with natural capabilities for abstract, conceptual thought, syntactical and propositional speech and intentional expression, it would be immoral to kill it. This would be an intelligent individual that might be a person such as are we, and to risk killing such being would be morally equivalent to risk killing a person, which would be unethical.

Tooley's theory of personhood is ambiguous and purely formal. The standard he proposes that an individual have a capability to desire to live is also quite vague and one has to wonder how the presence of this desire would be investigated. Virtually everyone has some desire to live as is seen by the fact that virtually all desire to sustain their lives by nourishment and hydration. One

[69] *Ibid*. Pp. 64-5. See Singer, Peter. *Practical Ethics*. (New York: Cambridge University Press, 1979) P. 117.

[70] Tooley, M. *Op. cit.*

[71] *Ibid*. P. 61.

wonders if Tooley demands that individuals verbally express their desire for it to be considered a legitimate desire? Does Tooley only want to allow voiced persons who can stand up and defend their rights to live full personhood, or does he think that the voiceless too have a desire to live that is sufficient?

Tooley's criteria for personhood are also exceedingly subjective. He implies that only those who have a concept of themselves as being a continuing subject are persons, but one must ask if he means this to be applied in a nondiscriminatory way to the mentally handicapped? It is by no means clear that these individuals have such a concept, and yet it is difficult to believe that they are not human persons. He claims that personhood requires a concept of the self as a continuing entity, but what this means is in no way self-evident. What does he mean when he says that the person must be conceived of as the continuing subject of experiences and desires? There are many individuals with serious mental handicaps and disabilities who might not have a concept of their selves perduring over time and being the continuing subject of experiences and emotions. Should they be denied the ascription of personhood? Tooley fails to see that the person is the principle that causes the existence and development of human material states and states of mind. The person is not simply identified with psychological operations or psychological states, but is the principle of human mental and bodily states. The person is not simply the concatenation of human states of mind or bodily states, but is the cause of those states. The person or soul is a compound individual that causes these and owns these two states, and does not emerge into full existence as these states do, but preexists and causes their emergence. There is not a succession of souls that first causes animal and material reality and existents to develop and then another soul that causes personal existents and actions to occur. Rather there is one soul, principle or person that exists and that causes the various material states and states of mind to exist and to develop.

The difficulty with his criteria is that his net is too fine and he casts it too widely. Tooley wants to only permit the killing of unborn and newly born disabled children, but his criteria would permit the killing of many more human beings than these. Probably the vast majority of children under seven do not have a concept of an enduring self that is the subject of experiences, and are therefore not yet persons. If having a "desire" to live is a necessary condition for being a person, it would seem that the comatose, suicidal, depressed, despairing, demented, many emotionally disturbed individuals and some severely brain-damaged patients could also be considered less than human. These classes of patients would seem to fit well into his category of "de-personed" human beings or humanoid animals. Tooley's definition of personhood is too narrow because it would exclude a large percentage of the very young and the very old from that category. It is a prescription for widespread nonvoluntary mercy killing of the handicapped and disabled of all ages.

## CONCLUSION

In its 1987 "Instruction on Respect for Human Life in its Origins and on the Dignity of Procreation: Replies to Certain Questions of the Day", issued by the Sacred Congregation for the Doctrine of the Faith, it was held that unborn human life should be regarded as if it were a person from conception onwards.[72] The aim of this chapter has been to show that there are sound philosophical reasons for making a presupposition of personhood of unborn human life and serious philosophical and logical problems in denying such a presupposition. This is not to say that it is absolutely certain that a person exists from conception onwards, but only that such a presupposition is not wholly groundless. The strongest argument for its personhood is the fact that denying its personhood commits one to holding a succession of souls theory and a biological class transfer if personhood is only acquired later on. Developmental theories of personhood fail to explain the nature of the causal agency that effects the development of the individual. These theories fail to see if the person develops along with the biological development of the individual, then there is no intrinsic agent to cause the development of the individual.

---

[72] Sacred Congregation for the Doctrine of the Faith, "Instruction on Respect for Human Life in Its Origins and on the Dignity of Procreation: Replies to Certain Questions." Part I, Sect. 1. 7.

# CHAPTER TWO
# THE MORALITY OF ABORTION: FACING THE ARGUMENTS

In a recent book, Beverly Wildung Harrison has argued that direct abortion might not destroy a being of significant moral value.[1] And in a pair of articles, "A Defense of Abortion" and "Rights and Death", Judith Jarvis Thomson claimed that there was neither a clear obligation or duty for a mother to sustain her unborn child nor that abortion would not always and everywhere be immoral.[2] Their views should be challenged because they present the most articulate and eloquent defenses of the "right to abortion" yet to be published. These arguments should be challenged, for if they can be successfully overcome, some of the strongest philosophical foundations for a right to abortion itself could be undermined.

In what follows, I wish to first show the transcendental value of the human person. It is necessary to do this to show the profound malice of abortion. Thomson objects to the claims that direct and deliberate killing of the unborn is always and everywhere wrong, but she does not show an understanding of what it is about the human person that gives it such value.[3] Then I will consider the arguments made in behalf of the permissibility of direct killing by Thomson. Further, I wish to suggest that Thomson does not believe the principles she has enunciated which permit abortion because they also permit actions to which she herself would object. She has neglected or misunderstood some fundamental moral principles and that her tolerance of abortion forces her to tolerate other kinds of killing she would not wish to permit.

---

[1] Harrison, Beverly, Wildung; *Our Right to Choose*, (Boston: Beacon Press, 1983).

[2] Thomson, Judith, Jarvis, "A Defense of Abortion" in *The Rights and Wrongs of Abortion*, (Princeton: Princeton University Press, 1974), pp. 3-23; and "Rights and Death", *Ibid.*, pp. 114-129.

[3] Thomson, "Rights and Death", pp. 120-121.

## A
## THE HUMAN PERSON: A BEING OF MORAL WORTH

Beverly Wildung Harrison asks in her book *Our Right to Choose* what the value of an unborn human being is.[4] This is a legitimate question because the strong anti-abortion argument is based on the view that the individual killed in abortion has such radical and extreme value that it deserves absolute protection from direct killing. What is it that gives this being such transcendent and radical value? Why do we commonly say that a human person is of greater value than is any other individual object? Paul Ramsey has argued that the person possess an "untouchability", and that any unconsented touchings are a violation of the integrity of the person.[5] Why would he say this, and why do we say that no concatenation of objects can equal or surpass the value of a given individual human person?

In answer to these questions, William E. May denied the claim of Philip Wylie that the conceptus was "protoplasmic rubbish" and he has argued eloquently that the human person is a being of moral worth, a spiritual being that is different in kind from all other material beings.[6] I wish to affirm what May claims and show that from both the philosophical and theological perspectives that there are sound reasons for holding that the human person possesses a transcendent value that is distinct from the value of all other material creatures.

---

[4] Harrison, "Our Right to Choose", p. 207-8.

[5] Ramsey, Paul. *The Patient as Person*, (New Haven: Yale University Press, 1970), pp. 27-40.

[6] Philip Wylie, *The Magic Animal*, (New York: Doubleday: 1968, p. 272. William E. May notes that this passage is particularly virulent and filled with very strong invective against the sanctity of life. See his: *Human Existence, Medicine and Ethics*, (Chicago: Franciscan Herald Press, 1977) p. 108.

1. What gives objects or individuals their value is their capacity to actualize higher orders of value, meaning or logic.[7] For example, a supercomputer is of more value than is a stone because it is capable of giving existence to higher orders of value and meaning. The capacity to actualize the transcendent, more complex and higher orders or meaning logic and value is what gives it value.

In this perspective, it can be seen why the human person possesses a value that transcends that of other entities in the world.[8] The human person alone in the material universe is able to generate transcendent orders of value, logic, meaning in the world. Because of innate human capabilities of abstract, conceptual thought, intentional expression and syntactical and propositional speech, the human person can generate higher orders of logic, meaning, order and value. Without the human person, there would only be evolution, but no true history or no generation of the truly new and unique in creation, history and time. If higher orders of meaning, value and logic are generated in the material universe, it is because of the agency of human intelligence, insight and thought. Beings that have only capacities for conceptual thought and that lack capacities for human intentional expression generate orders of value, logic and meaning, but they do not compare to the complexity and order of those generated by human persons.

Human persons are beings of moral worth because they are the independent active causal agents responsible for the generation of these orders. Their value is different from that of other individuals because they are the prime creators of transcendent

---

[7] This is the fundamental question posed by the field of axiology, but its relevance here is primarily ethical. The question being faced is not why such nonhuman objects as rocks, telephones or angel food cakes have value, but rather why a serious moral violation occurs when an entity such as a human being is destroyed. See: Lonergan, S.J., Bernard. *Insight: A Study of Human Understanding*, (London: Longmans, 1957) Pp. 470-472.

[8] This point has been made by philosophers and theologians who point out that human freedom and intelligence are the cause of what is distinctively new in the universe. The capacity of human conceptual thought to generate what is truly new is seen most baldly in scientific discovery, but it is also evident in social structures, cultural patterns and speculative and abstract thought. See: Grisez, Germain. *The Way of the Lord Jesus*, (Chicago: Franciscan Herald Press, 1983) P. 238.

values in the material world. The person's role, function and operation is different from that of other material individuals in the created order, and this is the ground of its unique value. Persons are not simply objects that possess a set and fixed particular value themselves identical to that of other material individuals, but are the creators of higher values and of the material objects that possess higher value in the natural order. The value of the human person is seen in the fact that it is the being who actively creates objects of higher value, which manifests a capacity that is of greater value than are the values that are in fact created. Thus, a designer of computers is of more value than are computers, for the machines are mere reflections of the intelligence and creative capabilities of the designer. Similarly, products of human creative activity are but reflections of human creative genius.

2. The transcendent value of the human person is also seen in the very nature of the human person itself. According to classical views, the person is unique in the universe because it alone is composed of and integrates into one entity all of the basic elements of the world.[9] The person was traditionally conceived of as the pinnacle of creation because all of the elements of the natural order are found in the person. In the human person there are found mineral, vegetative, animal and spiritual elements united into the most complex living organism in the natural order. The specific and precise composition of these elements is not fully clear, but the doctrine of the supremacy of the human person in creation is an ancient one that has been repeatedly affirmed in contemporary philosophical and theological thought.

This transcendent value of the human person is also manifested by the fact that contemporary scientific thought asserts that biologically, the human being is the most complex animal in creation. The human brain, for example, is vastly more complex

---

[9] See: Sullivan, John: *The Image of God*. (Dubuque: Priory Press, 1964) for a very comprehensive study of the nature and value of the human person. Like most Christian authors, Sullivan grounds the value of the human person in the *imago Dei*, but Sullivan shows that philosophers saw radical value in the human person that was not grounded on the image of God.

than the brain of any other animal.[10] And while there are many similarities between the human person and other creatures, the human person is also strikingly different. And there are many behavior patterns of the human person that are strikingly different from those of other creatures.[11]

In the Christian perspective, the human person has dominion over creation because the person is the pinnacle of creation.[12] This supremacy does not justify a moral right to exploit the universe without restraint, but it does justify a right and duty to use the natural order for the true welfare and the common good of the human community. It also signifies the proximity of the human person to God, who is the creator and Lord of the universe. The person has been conceived of in the classical Christian era as the ambassador of God in the material world, and hence shared somewhat in the power, nature, order and wisdom of God.[13]

3. The human person is also considered to be of transcendent value in comparison to other creatures or beings because of the person's relationship to God. Classical orthodox Christian theology taught that the human person was spiritual in

---

[10] See: Ashley, O.P., Benedict; and O'Rourke, O.P., Kevin, *Health Care Ethics*, (St. Louis, 1981.) P. 307.

[11] See: Adler, Mortimer. *The Difference of Man and the Difference It Makes*. (Cleveland: Meridian Books, 1968). Pp.99-112. Adler makes the point that there are certain activities commonly performed by human beings that are different in kind from the actions of others. He also suggests that speech is unique to the human species, and I would add that such activities as worship, promise making, and vows in marriage or religious life are unique to human persons. Specifically, he mentions abstract thought, which is correlative to Aristotle's contemplation. See: J.L. Austin's *How To Do Things With Words*, (Cambridge: Harvard University Press, 1975, 2nd ed.) In addition, See: G.E.M. Anscombe, *Intention*, (New York: Cornell University Press, 1976) because it shows the intricacy of intentional action and from it we can draw the conclusion that these sorts of actions cannot be duplicated by other creatures.

[12] See: Maloney, S.J., George. *Man: The Divine Icon*, (Pecos: Mexico, 1973). Pp. 35, 55-57.

[13] *Ibid.*

nature and was thus the "imago Dei", the image of God.[14] There was much debate through early Christian history concerning the precise character of this notion, but the existence of the image of God in the human person has been repeatedly affirmed by many of the Fathers and Doctors of the Church.[15]

Precisely what the nature of this image is in the person is not clear, but it was evident to the early Fathers and Doctors that the person in some way mirrors or images God because among all material creatures, the person is capable of love and of free moral action, and is spiritual in essence.[16] All of this is possible because of the spiritual nature of the person, and the orthodox Christian tradition claimed that the person participated or shared in the divine nature.[17] This should not be construed in pantheistic terms, but as merely holding that the human person represented or mirrored the divine presence in the material world. This notion has its roots in pagan thought and philosophy, but it was incorporated into Trinitarian thought and did not jeopardize any fundamental Christian doctrines.[18] It is this nature which links the human

---

[14] See: Sullivan, O.P., *The Image of God*; and Crouzel, S.J., Henri, *Theologie de l'Image de Dieu chez Origene*, (Paris: Aubier, 1955) for comprehensive studies of the classical doctrines of *imago Dei*.

[15] See: Maloney, S.J. *Man: The Divine Image*. He rightly suggests that imago Dei theology was much more typical of eastern theology than of Western thought, primarily because of eastern emphasis on the divinization of the human person rather than on sanctification. P. xi.

[16] *Ibid.* Pp. 187-198.

[17] Clement of Alexandria, *Stromata*. II, Ch. 19, P. 370. See generally: Burghardt, Walter, *The Image of God in Man According to Cyril of Alexandria*. (Washington: Catholic University of America Press, 1957); Leys, Roger. *L'image de Dieu chez Saint Gregoire de Nysse*, (Paris: Cerf, 1951); Lot-Borodine, M. "La Doctrine de la Deification chez Peres grecs", in *Revue de Histoire des Religions*, Tome 63, 1932.

[18] The closest that Christianity came to the pagan conceptions of *imago Dei* were in the Christian Gnosticism of Clement of Alexandria where assimilation to God was stressed, but in Trinitarian rather than in pantheistic terms. For a comparison of Christian and non-Christian developments of the *imago Dei* theme, see: Danielou, J. *Platonisme et Theologie Mystique: Doctrine Spirituelle de St. Gregoire de Nysse*, (Paris: Aubier, 1944). Also see: Plato, *Theatetus*, 176, B; *Timaeus*, 92,C; *Parmenides*, 132 C.

person to God most intimately and which makes the human person the "ambassador" of God.[19]

Implied by this doctrine of the person is the view that any directly lethal action against an innocent human person is in some fashion an action taken against God. By deliberately attaching such radical value to a human person, one was in an indirect and remote fashion attacking God because the person was the ambassador or legate of the divine and spiritual in the material world.[20]

4. The human person is a being of transcendent value, because it is the only free moral agent in the material world. That the human person is a free agent as is seen by the fact that the person's moral decisions are not *determined* by any extrinsic forces.[21] These decisions can be conditioned by various historical, social, cultural and familial factors, but the moral decisions of individuals are not determined.

That the human person is also a "moral" individual is seen by the fact that the person's moral identity is determined by the sorts of moral choices made by the person.[22] The human person alone is concerned with issues of justice, truth, religion, aesthetics, recreation, freedom, community and love, and it is this concern that marks the human person as unique and distinctive. A person acquires an identity as a murderer or thief, for example, by the moral character of the action he or she performs. These choices are freely made and when consent is given, the value of the action

---

[19] Maloney, *op. cit.* Pp. 49-51, 94. This theme is found throughout the Fathers, and Maloney notes that it takes a very explicit form in Ireneus and Athanasius.

[20] Genesis 9:6. Early authors drew a comparison between the image of a king or emperor struck on a coin and of the human person as an image of God. To deface the image of the emperor was equivalent to attacking him in person, just as to day burning a nation's flag is symbolically equivalent to attacking a nation.

[21] The freedom of the human person is affirmed in many philosophical works. For example, see: Grisez, Germain; Tollefson, Olaf; and Boyle, Joseph. *Free Choice: A Self-Referential Argument.* (Notre Dame: University of Notre Dame Press, 1976). P. 11. They affirm that a choice is free if the causal conditions are such that they would also be the causal conditions for not making the choice except insofar as these conditions include the person's very choosing itself and the consequences of his choice.

[22] William E. May, *Human Existence, Medicine and Ethics*, pp. 9-10.

chosen by the person is integrated by the person, which forms the moral character of the person.[23]

The human person is a free moral agent because its nature is spiritual and not wholly bound by the constraints of matter.[24] This spiritual nature is the source of the natural human capacities for intentional expression, abstract thought and syntactical and propositional speech. Because of the spiritual nature of the person, it is a being of a different order than are other material beings, and it can appropriately be called a being of "worth" rather than value.

The value of material individuals without moral capabilities is a sort of value that in some instances can be negotiated and balanced off against the value of other individuals in most circumstances without compromising morality. But persons must be treated differently from other individuals because the nature of the value of the person is different. This distinctive value and worth of the person, however, is that the person exists in the moral order while other creatures do not and this distinctive value justifies an absolute prohibition against deliberate and direct killing innocent human beings. Because other material individuals do not exist in the moral order and do not have the moral rights that persons have, they can be placed in the service of the morally legitimate needs of the human person.[25] We attribute value to those individuals, but I wish to suggest that ascribing moral worth to a human being is more appropriate. By this I would affirm with Paul Ramsey that the person is a being that is to be regarded differently from other entities, is untouchable and exists at a different order of value than do other individuals. The person is the evaluator of the material

---

[23] *Ibid.* P. 121. May correctly points out that our motives do not disclose our moral identity as well as do our actions. Actions do this because they reveal choices which is not so clearly the case when dealing purely with motives or intentions.

[24] See: Ashley, O.P., Benedict; and O'Rourke, O.P., Kevin. *op. cit.* Pp. 32-3. Also see: Maloney, *op. cit.* P. 8.

[25] For alternative views, see: Singer, Peter, *Practical Ethics*, (New York: Cambridge, 1979.) 117-25. Singer argues that because some animals have more capabilities for certain sorts of actions at birth that they have more rights than do newborn infants. He justifies infanticide by arguing that just as it would not be immoral to kill some monkeys at birth, it would not be immoral to kill some infants because they are of less value than are some monkeys.

universe because it stands in a superior position to the universe. The person ascribes value to other beings, and determines the standards of value for the rest of the material universe.

## B
## GIVING MATERNAL SUPPORT TO THE UNBORN

In her articles, Judith Jarvis Thomson makes a number of different arguments to justify abortion which must be challenged. First, she suggests there would be nothing wrong with a woman disconnecting a terminally ill world-famous violinist who temporarily needed to use her body to recover from a disease and who had been attached to her without her knowledge or consent, thereby causing his death.[26] Because of this, Thomson argues that there would be nothing wrong with an abortion as this is morally identical to a mother "disconnecting" her unborn child from a woman as the woman disconnects the violinist.[27]

But in fact, these actions are quite different. The violinist is connected to the woman without her consent and his willful remaining there is a deliberate action that is against her rights. The violinist's being attached to her is a clear case of unconsented surgery that is not in any therapeutic interest to the mother. The unborn child, however, is not illegitimately connected to the woman by an unconsented nontherapeutic medical procedure. Thus, disconnecting the violinist and not removing the unborn child are both morally justified because they are different kinds of acts. Thomson's argument fails because there are significant differences between abortion and the hypothetical situation she proposes, and there are a number of faults with her analogy that must be pointed out.

1. She assumes that the support a mother gives to her unborn child is analogous to a medical treatment which can be withdrawn when it becomes too burdensome for the mother.[28] But

---

[26] Thomson, "A Defense of Abortion", pp. 4-5.

[27] Ibid. P. 4.

[28] Ibid. P. 13.

if what the mother does for an unborn child is a medical treatment, it is a very peculiar kind of medical treatment. For the mother does not cure, remedy or palliate any clinical diagnosable condition of the unborn child, and hence what she provides is not a medical treatment as are other kinds of treatment. In recent decades this misunderstanding of the nature of medical treatments has expanded widely such that virtually anything done to support the life of another seems to be a medical treatment. Thomson misconstrues abortion to be simply an omission of an action, when it is in fact a deliberate action taken against the life of the unborn child. If abortion is an omission of maternal support, then why has it traditionally required specialized medical skills to perform it? Granting legal permission for this sort of action compromises laws prohibiting lethal actions taken by private citizens against other innocent private citizens.

The mother in fact is not providing any therapeutic treatments for the child. The means by which the life of the child is supported is not strictly comparable to a therapeutic act undertaken by a health care provided, but one is only a natural measure of protecting and sustaining the life of the child. The violinist is suffering from a clinically diagnosable pathological condition and he is supported by a medical treatment attaching him to the woman against her rights. But the child is not suffering from any such pathology, and it does not need the medical treatments that the violinist needs to survive. If the violinist were to be separated from the woman, he would die from an underlying pathological condition and not from a withdrawal of medical treatment. But if the child were to die, it would be because it was denied natural life support and protection. Abortion is not the mere withdrawal of an extraordinary medical treatment because the withdrawal of maternal support creates a new and independent lethal cause is imposed on the child. Thomson has failed to see the difference between fetal euthanasia and the withdrawal of a medical treatment.

She argues that the mother "owns" the house in which the unborn child resides and the mother therefore has the right to drive out the child just as one would drive out a burglar.[29] The womb is

---

[29] *Ibid.* P. 10.

not a "jointly owned house" in her view, but is the sole possession of the mother. The use of claims, rights and titles to organs of the body is a peculiar way of expressing the relationship of the child to the mother.[30] But even if the mother is the sole "owner" of the house, does this mean that the unborn child is a "squatter" that can be expelled and even killed at her whim. Or is not the child a "temporary" dweller who at has a right not to be killed for being there? Thomson fails to see that the womb is the permanent possession of the mother but is also the temporary possession of the unborn child.[31] The fact that the mother has the natural capability in the first place to provide shelter for the unborn child suggests that the child has at least some claim to the womb.

Using Thomson's terminology, the child has no "claim" to the mother's fallopian tubes if being there would pose a serious threat to her health. Because of this, the child could be indirectly removed by direct removal of the tubes if its dislocation would pose an imminent lethal threat to the mother.[32] It is clear that the child has no title to the mother's heart, brain or stomach, as is seen by the fact that it would pose a serious health threat to the mother if the unborn child lodged there. But the child has a claim to the womb, because its presence there ordinarily causes no grave threat to the health of the mother in the absence of maternal defects and also because the uterus is ordered naturally to sustain the child. The unborn child is radically isolated from the mother in the womb,

---

[30] See: John Finnis, "The Rights and Wrongs of Abortion" in *The Rights and Wrongs of Abortion*. P. 91.

[31] Thomson, "A Defense of Abortion", p. 9. It is difficult to speak of "ownership" of human bodies or organs in any strict and unequivocal fashion, and to speak in this way might well unduly complicate the issue. The temporary claims of the unborn child to body of the mother does not mean that the claims of the child are wholly without merit for that temporary duration of time. One suspects that underlying her arguments about ownership of bodies is an argument that the claims made by the child to the time, energy and dedication of the mother to the child after the birth of the child is what is really at stake.

[32] This is admittedly a peculiar way of justifying indirect abortion to save the life of the mother, but the employment of the terminology and argument of Thomson's suggests a justification for limited indirect abortion when it alone will save the life of an innocent human being.

and even when the unborn child is severely handicapped and ill-formed, it does not ordinarily pose a serious threat to the mother there. The fact that the child does not ordinarily pose a lethal threat to the mother in the womb suggests that the child does have some sort of rightful claim to the womb.

If burden is the critical factor justifying aborting unborn children, it would also seem to be the critical factor in infanticide because there is no significant difference between unborn and newly born children. If a mother can withdraw maternal support from an unborn child because of the burden involved, then she should be able to withdraw it from a newborn handicapped child when such a child imposes equal or greater burdens on her. Thomson has unwittingly endorsed neonatal infanticide by omission by her teachings, and her principles permit at the speculative level eugenic medicine by arguing that the mother has no duty to give support to the unborn child because her burdens increase after birth.

2. Thomson implicitly believes that the fetus is either a formal or a material aggressor against the mother. If the unborn child is a formal aggressor, then there would probably be no profound moral problem with the mother killing the child. But if the child is neither a formal aggressor at all, or is only a material aggressor, it would be difficult to justify directly killing it. It is hard to see how the unborn child is even a material aggressor, for the normal threats to maternal health come from the inadequacies or defects of the mother more often than from any action or condition of the unborn child. As was said above, the child is so isolated from the mother by the placenta that it is seldom the case that the child *itself* is a threat to the mother.

If the fetus were to be a threat to the mother, then it would only be a material and not a formal threat because of its inability to perform free, knowing and intentional actions, and it is not permissible to directly kill it as a material aggressor. For example, if a party of potholers was trapped in a flooding cave because the leader of the party was stuck in the mouth of the cave, it would not be permissible to blow him out of the hole with explosives. To do this would be to cause his death as an immoral means to achieve a morally good end.[33] If a trolley driver lost its brakes while going down a steep mountain side and had to choose between turning at a fork in the tracks to the left where there is a baby or to the right where there is a group of armed people, theoretically it could turn either way without violating justice because of the total absence of freedom.[34] Similarly, one would not be morally justified in not directly killing an unborn child because it is not a formal aggressor, just as the trolley driver and person stuck in the mouth of the cave are not formal aggressors.

Thomson compares the relationship of the unborn child to the mother to that of Smith having Jones' coat which Jones needs to survive.[35] She claims that Jones could take the coat away by force, and implicitly holds that Smith has no right to the coat, which is a doubtful analogy to the relationship of the mother and child. But in doing this, she reduces the mother-child relationship to a purely consensual one and this denies that the child has any natural right to his or her parents. One would wonder if she would contend as well that the services a mother offers her child are purely consensual, or if the child has a right to those services. If an Afghan parent agrees that her child should be taken to Moscow for five years of political indoctrination, does the child have any natural right not to be taken from his or her family? It would seem that Thomson would have to say that the child does not. The difficulty is that this is not truly analogous to the relationship of the mother and child. It would be a closer analogy if Smith and Jones jointly owned the coat and both equally needed it. It would be a closer analogy to compare it to a situation where two men needed a life raft to survive, for in this case, neither could push the other off to save their lives because both have an equal right to the raft and the

---

[33] It might be argued that the death of the man was not the means by which the party was saved, and that the means used was the explosion employed to enlarge the hole so that the party could escape. But if that is true, then why were not the explosives placed where they would not injure the man. The man had to die for them to live, and this makes his death a means to an end. This is an instance of the Caiaphas principle asserting the legitimacy of killing an innocent to protect the many. See: Philipa Foot, "The Problem of Abortion and the Doctrine of Double Effect" *Oxford Review* 5, 1967, pp. 5-15.

[34] *Ibid.*

[35] Thomson, "A Defense of Abortion", p. 9-10.

raft not be the sole possession of either man. To use Thomson's analogy, neither Jones nor Smith have a clear and uncontested title to the coat, and thus the comparison is not entirely convincing. These cases do not justify direct abortion and they only suggest that neither the mother nor the unborn child can be directly killed if their lives are threatened.

Thomson also cites the implausible case of a woman trapped in a house with a rapidly growing child to justify direct abortion.[36] Extrapolating from this example, she argues that direct abortion can be morally justified because material aggressors can be directly and willfully killed. Again, using such hypothetical or science fiction cases is a weak way to argue for a point. But granting that this is true, let us turn the tables and ask if the adult could be killed if the child was the one who was being threatened, for it would seem that the child would have the dominant right to life and that the adult could be killed. Thus, if an unborn child found itself being threatened because of a pathology in the mother, Thomson's logic would compel her to admit that the mother would then have to be killed rather than the child.

Thomson has not proven her case that material aggressors can be directly killed. The situation where the mother's life is in danger because of pregnancy is more like a situation where a child sets a car unintentionally in motion while playing in it, causing it to threaten to run over another. It would not be morally legitimate to shoot the child as the car and not the child is the real threat. Similarly, in abortion, the child himself is not the threat, and it cannot be intentionally killed for an action it did not intentionally perform.

A crucial flaw with her argument is that she does not distinguish the condition of pregnancy from the existence of the unborn child. Most of the burdens which she seeks to protect the mother from are caused by the pregnancy rather than by the child or by any deliberate actions of the child. Because of this, it is not clear that the child can be legitimately killed on account of conditions that the child did not create. If the child were the cause of the pregnancy, it *might* be morally permissible *at the speculative level* to end its life, but that is not the case, as the child is the

---

[36] *Ibid.* P. 8.

product of the action of the mother.

3. Thomson justifies abortion because of the burden imposed on the mother.[37] But because there are lower levels of medical care available to poorer women, this principle would give them a stronger right to abortion than would be had by women of greater means, which would be discriminatory. This is a justifiable conclusion to be drawn from her principles even though it is discriminatory and eugenic because it justifies and facilitates eliminating the poorer classes in society.

Thomson proves too much by arguing that the mother is permitted to "withdraw maternal support" from an unborn child if this support proves to be unduly burdensome for her. For, if what the mother does to support an unborn child is an extraordinary and morally elective action, then a mother could equally "withdraw maternal support" from a child after birth in many cases. The mother provides shelter and nourishment for the unborn child, and if she could be permitted to "withhold" that from an unborn child, she could then "withdraw" this from newly born infants and starve, dehydrate and expose them after birth. This could be justified because there is often more burden for the mother in caring for children after birth than in gestating them before birth. It is to be doubted, however, that Thomson would agree to this even though her principles commit her to this conclusion. Her principle would permit neonatal euthanasia because the burden of postnatal care is often greater than that of prenatal care. Also, it would be justified in her view because the rights of a newly born child are not significantly greater than those of a late-term unborn baby, and the mother would have a stronger right to withdraw her support from them than from the unborn child. This can be argued because gestation does not require the deliberate acts of providing nutrition, protection from exposure, and sanitary care that are required after birth.

Thomson denies that withdrawing maternal support is a form of direct killing by omission because the burdens of pregnancy can be so great that pregnancy cannot be required in justice.[38] The

---

[37] *Ibid.* Pp. 17-21.

[38] Thomson, "A Defense of Abortion", p. 17.

question of whether pregnancy is *unjustly* burdensome is a most difficult one, but some considerations are in order. For the woman to whom pregnancy poses no lethal threats, it is hard to see how it could be so burdensome that ending the life of the child can be justified. If caring for the child is so radically burdensome that it could not be required by justice, it would be hard to require caring for infants, incompetent handicapped individuals or elderly persons as well. If pregnancy presents life-threatening burdens, justice would not be violated if the pregnancy was ended, even if this meant that the life of the child would be indirectly ended.

A basic problem with Thomson's argument from burdensomeness is that its vagueness places the handicapped and incompetent in jeopardy of abuse, neglect, and discrimination. For if the support commonly required of a mother for her child is radically burdensome, it is hard to see how supporting the disabled and incompetent could be required in justice as a matter of duty or obligation.

Thomson argues that pro-lifers who permit abortion in the case of rape but not in other instances are being inconsistent because the quality of the action by which the child is created should not influence the morality of the act of killing the child.[39] In saying this she is correct, and that is why not all pro-lifers would permit abortion in the case of rape. The child generated from rape is an innocent victim of the rapist, just as is the mother, and if child can be killed it would seem that the mother could be as well.

4. She argues that abortion is morally equivalent to withdrawal of maternal support.[40] But if what is done in an abortion is merely the "withdrawal of maternal support", what would constitute active and positive, direct killing of the unborn? She has mischaracterized abortion as an omission or withdrawal of support, for it rather seems to be a positive and deliberate physical act taken to destroy the unborn child. When an abortion is performed, the child does not die from some underlying pathological condition, but from the new and independent lethal treat posed by the abortive actions. The act by which "support" is withdrawn from an unborn

---

[39] *Ibid.* P. 5.

[40] *Ibid.*

child is more like a craniotomy than anything else, and certainly a craniotomy would be active killing. She implies that there is no difference between unplugging a violinist and an abortion, but she ignores some crucial differences between these two sorts of actions.[41] When one unplugs a violinist, one does not cut away living tissue as one does in abortion, and abortions are much more grisly than is a mere unplugging of a tube used to sustain another's life. Abortions involve burning the skin off the child with salt solution, dismembering the child, or violently expelling the child from the womb. Unplugging the violinist is actually more akin to removing a respirator, and that sort of action does not involve immediate physical assault on the individual as does abortion.

If what the abortionist does is actually like "withdrawal of maternal support", one would have to ask why the woman could not imitate that act and simply reach over and strangle the violinist, for abortion is more like that than it is like removing sophisticated medical treatment. The violinist's right to use the woman's body may be in doubt, but it seems clear that he has a right not to be stabbed or dismembered by another, which is actually what occurs in an abortion. The difference between withdrawing a tube or other medical devices and an abortion is also symbolized rather clearly in the emotional reactions of nursing and abortion personnel, for there is a much higher "burn out" rate among abortion personnel than there is among nursing population at large.[42] She fails to see that abortion is more akin to cutting off a man's hands who is clinging to a life raft than to the mere "withdrawal of maternal life support". It is a bloody affair conducted on a person who is not terminally ill, imminently dying or suffering from any clinically diagnosable pathological condition, unlike the violinist. The child's life is strong

---

[41] *Ibid*. P. 22. She claims that it is permissible to withdraw "maternal support" from an unborn child because a woman would be permitted to withdraw support from the violinist. But she says that she could not reach around and slit the violinist's throat. But what she fails to see is that abortion is more akin to slitting a throat than it is to merely disconnecting a tube. Nowhere does Thomson actually describe what is involved in an abortion, but the enduring impression is given that it involves little more than withdrawing a respirator rather than the violent dismemberment of the child.

[42] Tredgold, R. F., "Psychiatric Indications for Termination of Pregnancy", *Lancet*, 2 (1964) P. 1253. Also see: Jeffcoate, T. N. A., "Indications for Therapeutic Abortion", *Clinical Obstetrics and Gynecology*, 7, (March 1964) P. 52.

and just beginning, and abortion ends it.  But the violinist's life is weak, failing and ending and can probably be sustained only for a short period of time.

5. Thomson denies assertions that "no one may choose" to directly, freely and deliberately kill one innocent person rather than another, and she asserts that it is morally permissible to decide which of two innocent persons might be deliberately killed in some circumstances.[43]  One may choose to avoid killing one innocent person rather than another, but one may not choose to directly, deliberately, and willfully kill one rather than the other.  For as mentioned above one can choose to turn a trolley that is careening out of control down a hill to kill one person rather than another, but this is more of a choice to avoid killing one person rather than to directly kill.  And in this situation, the choice of the one who does the actual killing must be to avoid killing rather than to choose to kill one person rather than the other.

Thomson admits that an individual does not have the right to defend his life by torturing another innocent person if he is threatened with death by a third party for not doing so.[44]  But, according to her, it is legitimate for a mother to abort the unborn child if it threatens her life.  She claims that the situations are different because in the former case both persons are threatened, while in the latter, only the mother is threatened.[45]  But she does not see that the threat being posed by the unborn child is not an intentional threat, and that the child itself might not be the cause of the threat and that the case is different because of this.  The threat by the one being tortured against the other is made under duress and is not a fully formal threat.  Because of this, the threat posed is really closer to being a material threat than it is to a formal threat.  Thomson permits direct killing when there is only a material threat at best, and one wonders why she doesn't allow it

---

[43] *Ibid.* Pp. 9-10.

[44] *Ibid.* P. 9.

[45] *Ibid.* P. 9.

when the threat is formal but done under duress.[46] Thomson would not allow deliberate killing when a person is forced to threaten and the formal threat is not free, yet she will allow it when a material threat is posed that is free.

Thomson wants to know what the difference is between aborting when a child threatens the life of the mother and disconnecting the violinist, for she believes that if aborting to save the mother is permissible then disconnecting the violinist should be as well.[47] Permissible abortion, even when the mother is lethally threatened, involves an action which immediately and proximately removes the threat, and remotely threatens the life of the child. But disconnecting the violinist involves immediately killing the violinist when a threat is not posed. If the violinist posed a lethal threat to the mother, it would be permissible to disconnect him.

## C
## GOOD AND MINIMALLY DECENT SAMARITANISM

Thomson wonders if a woman can voluntarily put an end to what she has voluntarily brought into existence, and she suggests that this cannot be done without any significant qualifications.[48] This possibility needs to be examined closely, however, for the child is not the product solely of the mother, but is also the product of the father and of society as well. The child has obligations to people other than the parents, and it must fulfill those as well. Thomson complains about complete prohibitions of abortion by claiming that laws supporting this view demand that women not be just "Minimally Decent Samaritans" but that they be Good Samaritans.[49] In saying this, she means that laws today require women to do far

---

[46] *Ibid*. P. 22. She allows the violinist to be killed by unplugging and an unborn child to be killed when it poses a "threat". But neither of these threats are deliberate and intentional. One has to wonder what sort of violence she would permit in the event of intentional threats.

[47] Thomson, "Rights and Deaths, p. 117.

[48] *Ibid*. Pp. 11, 20.

[49] *Ibid*. Pp. 18-22.

more to protect the lives of unborn children than is demanded to protect the lives of others in morally similar situations. Because of this, the rights and powers of the parents of the child are not unlimited.

    1. In the case of rape, Thomson argues that the child has no right to use the mother's womb as the mother did not invite the child into the womb.[50] This is an interesting assertion because she has claimed elsewhere that the circumstances surrounding the placing of the child in the mother's womb should have no effect on the rights or duties of the child. It is also interesting because it suggests that people who swim for life boats could be deliberately killed by those in the boats to save their lives, or that people fleeing flood waters to the rooftops of others' houses could be directly killed because they too were not "invited".

    She argues that the child can be fittingly compared to a burglar who creeps into the woman's bedroom through the window despite bars she constructed to protect herself.[51] This comparison, however, is not an accurate portrayal of the relationship of the unborn child to mother because the burglar is a formal aggressor who obviously intends to do the woman harm. On the other hand, the child is, at worst, a material aggressor who does not formally intend harm. The rapist, rather than the unborn child is more aptly compared to the burglar because both are formal aggressors. The unborn child is more like a baby who is squeezed between the bars of the woman's room by someone else than to a burglar because the child is not a formal aggressor against the mother. The burglar would not be there if harm was not intended, but the unborn baby could easily be there without intending harm. Just as it would be an injustice to the baby put into the woman's bedroom by another, so also is it an injustice to kill unborn children through abortion.

    2. Because she regards the unborn child as an unjust aggressor, not only in cases of rape, but also when pregnancy is not desired, Thomson believes that it is excessively harsh to prohibit

---

[50] *Ibid.* P. 12.

[51] *Ibid.* Pp. 14-5.

abortion in all instances.[52] To justify this judgment, she compares the unborn child conceived against the wishes of the woman to a form of "people seeds" that implant in the carpets of the woman's home against her wishes.[53] Just as a tidy housekeeper would be justified to rid her house of these, so also would a woman be justified in ridding herself of unwanted unborn children. One wonders, however, if this doesn't demean the unborn child by comparing the child to refuse, pests or litter that any decent person would wish to banish. There also seems to be a significant difference between the ways in which a child enters a woman's life and the way in which the "people seeds" enter the woman's home. With the "people seeds", the woman takes no action that is naturally and inherently ordered toward human generation. For, depending on the company one keeps, opening windows does not usually cause one to become pregnant! Opening a window cannot be aptly compared to sexual relations or generating a child, for it is not naturally ordered to generation as is the sexual act. But with the generation of children, an action is taken that by its very nature is ordered to generating children. Thomson seems to think that pregnancy happens with complete inadvertence, as if it occurred when one backed into a Christmas tree.

In this example, Thomson suggests that pregnancy occurs as an unintended side effect of an action that was wholly oriented toward another end.[54] However, the very orientation and dynamism of sexual relations is both to unity of the partners and to the generation of a child. To say that pregnancy is a totally unintended and unforeseen consequence of sex relations is like saying that when one deliberately points a loaded pistol at another person and fires at point blank range the injury or death resulting is unforeseen and unintended. One cannot simply claim that one was launching a projectile in a given direction and that the injury or death of the person was not intended. For when one consents to the action, one consents to the entailed consequences of the action itself, as there

---

[52] *Ibid.* P. 15.

[53] *Ibid.* P. 15.

[54] *Ibid.* P. 15.

are certain effects of actions that are not only foreseen but entailed by an action and are intrinsic to the actions.[55] Pregnancy is an effect of an action to which one gives implicit consent, except when raped, when engaging in sexual relations just as one implicitly and conditionally consents to the death of another when one deliberately fires a pistol at them at point-blank range. Thomson denies that the intention of the action encompasses the intention of the agent, and because of this she believes that there is no duty not to kill the unborn child.

3. In order to argue that Good Samaritanism is too demanding Thomson claims that the child does not have a right to be in the mother.[56] This is doubtful, because the child's presence in the mother was the result of a free and deliberate action by the mother, and the child violates no duties to the mother by being there. She draws a strict analogy between the violinist and the unborn child, but she forgets that the woman does not have the moral duties toward the violinist as she would have to an unborn child because it was her action that brought the unborn child into existence. These duties flow from the fact that her actions brought the child into existence. If the child entered by womb by its own deliberate act, it could be argued that a duty not to be there had been violated. But as the child was placed there by another, it cannot be argued that the child violated a duty. It is legitimate for Thomson to say that the rapist or any other individual has no right to engage in sexual relations with her, but it is hard to validly claim that the unborn child violates a duty in being placed in the mother by another. For even in the case of rape, the child does not violate any duties by being placed in the woman.

In contrast to the unborn child, the violinist is attached to the mother by a choice of the Society of Music Lovers and they violate a duty not to impinge on the body of the woman. The violinist has an obligation to obtain the consent of the mother before being attached to her because he can give consent to his actions, while an unborn child cannot. A conclusion that can be drawn from

---

[55] This principle lies at the heart of the doctrine of double effect. See my "Stones and Streetcars: A Clarification of The Doctrine of Double Effect", *Irish Theological Quarterly*, 1981, pp. 127-136.

[56] *Ibid.* Pp. 20.

Thomson's analysis is that the unborn child would have to gain the explicit consent of the mother to assume residence in the mother. The violinist will be free to unplug himself and walk away, which the unborn child would not, and the Society of Music Lovers would also be free to remove him. If the violinist obtains her consent, it is by no means clear that the woman would then be totally free to disconnect him, but this is a hard question that Thomson does not confront. It would seem because of this that the aggressor against the mother would have more of a right to abort the woman than would the woman herself, because he implanted the child. The aggressor would have an obligation to abort the child, an obligation stronger than the mother's.

4. Thomson believes that direct killing can be as permissible as indirect killing in some cases, and she cites cases to prove this.[57] She calls the killing of children about to launch a missile in an unjust attack indirect, but the killing of children being trained to launch the missile is direct, even though she holds it to be permissible.[58] She claims that the former are innocent of unjust aggression, while the latter are not, and the former killing is direct while the latter is indirect killing.[59] This is a bad example to illustrate her principle that direct killing of the innocent is sometimes permissible, for the children in the latter group are remote threats while those in the former are proximate threats to the innocent. The proximate character of the children's threat would be more clearly seen if the children were presented as adults, for their lack of comprehension of what they do clouds the nature of their threat. In addition, Thomson fails to prove her point because both groups of children are threats and are therefore legitimate military targets. She is searching for an example of direct and indirect killing that clarifies the distinction but seems to be unable to find one, for in both cases, the killing is indirect, because both groups are formal threats, one immediate, and the other remote.

---

[57] Thomson, "Rights and Deaths", pp. 120-122.

[58] *Ibid.* Pp. 121-22.

[59] *Ibid.* P. 122.

Admitting that the unborn child can be killed unintentionally as a foreseen side-effect of a therapeutic act to save the life of the mother affirms that in some cases the unborn child is a "quasi-aggressor". But this is not to admit that direct and deliberate killing of the child in isolation from the therapeutic actions taken to save her life is morally permissible. This prohibition denies the mother the right to directly kill the child by an action that had no immediate therapeutic values an unintended consequence of the therapeutic action. Thomson objects to this tradition by saying that it requires mothers to be "Splendid Samaritans", but she fails to see that this view treats the mother and child as equals. This tradition prohibits removing the child while leaving the womb intact, or shucking out the child from a tubal pregnancy because it sees both the mother and the child as innocent and not as aggressors.

Thomson wants to understand the mother-child relationship in terms of burdens and rights, and it is not clear that this is the best way to understand this complex relationship.[60] If the relationship of mother to child was a therapeutic one, this model would be more fitting, but this is not the case by any means. Thomson forces us ask if the Good Samaritan-victim relationship should be understood in the context of burdens and benefits. There are relationships of care and nurture, and they are exemplified by the relationships of mother and child, Good Samaritan and victim. There are obligations to give care and nurture, comfort and feeding that are different from obligations to heal, and the benefit-burden model does not capture these obligations adequately. The Good Samaritan aided the victim, not because there was minimal burden involved in his aid, but because care, comfort and nurture are to be accorded to all as a simple matter of basic and natural justice.

5. Thomson wishes to repeal abortion laws because they are "Good Samaritan" laws and she believes that the should only require

---

[60] Finnis makes this point against Thomson and it is correct. The difficulty with analysis of abortion in terms of rights is that it fails to see that the child is very much a benefit to the mother. Because of this, a rights analysis demands that the benefits of the child must be compared to and balanced off against the burdens brought by the child, which is a very difficult if not impossible endeavor. See: Thomson, "Rights and Death", p. 114.

"Minimally Decent Samaritanism".[61]  But in urging this, she misconstrues the actions of the Good Samaritan to be heroic actions. Rather than being heroic, the Good Samaritan has merely done what is to be accorded to individuals as a matter of decency.[62] It is not so much that the Samaritan was good or splendid, but that the priest and Levite violated the basic norms of human decency by refusing to even provide food and shelter to the victim. If the parable of the Good Samaritan argues for anything, it argues for giving minimal care and treatment even for those with whom we have no special relationship to others. The Good Samaritan cares for an unknown victim of violence, and the parable argues for doing at least what he did for the children we conceive. There are certain bonds that unite us as human beings, and calling the maintenance of those bonds an extraordinary burden is to severely weaken those fundamental bonds.

Thomson's understanding of Good Samaritanism fails because it justifies not only abortion, but infanticide and mercy killing as well. If a mother can "withdraw" life support from an unborn baby because it is excessive and heroic, why cannot she withdraw even more troubling forms of care from newly born babies? And if the grisly bloody affair of abortion is a "medical treatment" that can be "withdrawn" when too burdensome, why could not a mother push her newborn child's head under the bath water because other forms or "care" were too "burdensome". After all, a newborn can impose more demands on a mother's time and energies than can an unborn baby in many circumstances. If mothers can forego these forms of care for unborn children, what is to stop children from withdrawing similar forms of "medical treatment" from their aging patients when it becomes "too burdensome"?

She claims that there should be obligations to preserve life only if those caring for the person have an interest in preserving the

---

[61] Thomson, "A Defense of Abortion", p. 19.

[62] That what the Good Samaritan did was an act of common decency and not a heroic act of life saving. That this is the case is seen by the fact that the Levite and priest are considered to be indecent for having done nothing. If what the Good Samaritan did was elective and not required by justice why then was there the subtle condemnation of the Levite and Priest, and why has not the Good Samaritan been considered through history as the "Splendid" Samaritan?

life or relationship to the person.[63] The point of the Good Samaritan parable seems to be that we have duties to preserve life even when we have no "interest" in doing so. Why do "interests" and relationships strengthen a duty to not deliberately kill? Does Thomson's principle that relationships make duties to protect life stronger mean that our obligations to the nameless starving of the world are diminished or nonexistent just because we have specific and precise relationship to them? Would not her principle imply that those with closer relationships would have stronger duties to preserve life? Would it not mean that a mother would have an almost absolute obligation to preserve the life of her unborn child? If a person who had no relationship to a baby who was drowning from a bathtub, would such an individual be free to not lift the baby's head from the water? Thomson fails to see that it is not the relationship that one has to another that grounds the duty to sustain life. Rather it is the capacity of the individual to sustain life with minimal risk and burden that makes it morally obligatory.

Thomson claims that she only wants to eliminate burdens to the woman and does not wish to have dead babies is empty, for there are certain burdens that can only be eliminated by the death of the baby.[64] It is not clear that she believes this, however, for if the baby is not dead, the mother would incur at least some responsibility for caring for and raising the child. To be totally free of burdens it would be necessary for the baby to die, and Thomson gives no indication that she would protest allowing this in some instances.

6. In her reply to the objections raised by John Finnis, Thomson argues that the innocence of the victims of lethal actions does not make the lethal actions direct or indirect.[65] She claims

---

[63] *Ibid.* P. 21.

[64] Thomson claims that she only wants to disconnect the violinist, but this is doubtful. It seems that she wants to relieve the mother of not just the burdens of pregnancy, but of parenting as well. It is doubtful that Thomson would agree that if the child could survive "disconnection" from the mother that she would compel the mother to parent the child. Thomson seems to implicitly hold that the unborn child must die because of her emphasis on the mother's right to be free from *any* unconsented burdens.

[65] Thomson, "Rights and Deaths", p. 123.

that there are many directly lethal actions taken against the innocent that are morally permissible.[66] Intentional and direct killing of the innocent is morally culpable, and she fails to see that her understanding places the innocent wholly at the mercy of aggressors. The only way of protecting the innocent from aggressors is by affirming that directly lethal action against a person occurs when the person killed is not a formal aggressor. If the "victim" is guilty of posing a formally lethal threat against another innocent person, the "victim" is an aggressor, and lethal action becomes direct. But if the victim does not pose such a threat, any lethal action posed against him is unjustly killing. If the innocence of the victim is not the criterion by which the permissibility of lethal actions was based, then what other basis could there be, given the fact that burden cannot be an adequate basis for determining justice.

Thomson suggests that Finnis would accept the use of some abortifacients because they are not as physically proximate in their mode of killing as are most abortion procedures.[67] This claim is questionable, however because these chemicals achieve the same effects in relation to the unborn child that the more physically proximate means do such as suction abortions. As a result, Finnis would probably be as critical of them as he is of the more proximate measures. Thomson claims that Finnis would object to a woman threatened by a pregnancy taking a medicine to cause a miscarriage in order to save her life because of the threat posed by her pregnancy.[68] She is not entirely correct in saying this, for if the woman took the medicine precisely to kill the baby, then her intention would be directly lethal against the child and morally unacceptable and it would seem that Finnis would undoubtedly object to that. But if she took the medicine to relieve the threat, and did not directly intend the death of the baby, it would be an indirect form of killing and permissible.

---

[66] *Ibid.*

[67] *Ibid.* Pp. 114-5.

[68] *Ibid.* P. 119.

## D
## THE RIGHT TO LIFE

1. Thomson suggests that the right to life is problematic and she asks what it means to have such a right.[69] She sees difficulties in the contention that the right to life imposes a duty on all to refrain from intentional lethal actions and omissions against the innocent. She seems to deny that directly lethal omissions can be equivalent to directly lethal commissions and that both can be forbidden by justice. She denies that it means that all must refrain from taking directly lethal actions against innocent persons. Because of the complexity of the right to life, she wonders if the range of our right to life is determined by the physical distance of the distance of those who can support life from those who are asserting their right.

Thomson claims that the strength of one's claims to life is dependent on the physical proximity of others, and she finds this shocking.[70] But, in claiming this, she caricatures the classical ordinary-extraordinary distinction and has shown that she fails to understand it. It is not distance that makes an action obligatory in justice, but whether or not exceptional trials must be borne and whether heroic fortitude is required to save one's life. She questions whether it means that one has a right to be given the bare minimum to survive, and she thus wonders if Henry Fonda has a moral duty to lay his soothing hand on her brow to save her life.[71] Her view suggests that the right to life is a limited right, one that is limited by the physical proximity of agents who can comply with one's demands for support. But that argues very strongly against morally indirect abortion, for if it were true that distance constituted duties to preserve life, then the mother would have the strongest duty to save the life of the child because she is closest to the child.

Nonetheless, it is true that the right to life should be

---

[69] Thomson, "A Defense of Abortion", p. 11.

[70] Ibid.

[71] Ibid.

properly specified, but this does not mean that one can simply say that the right to life does not permit directly lethal commissions or omissions. She objects to the view that the right to life permits the unborn child unlimited use of the woman's body.[72] This, however, is not the case, for as mentioned above, the right to life of the child is limited if the pregnancy threatens the life of the mother. In that case, therapeutic action to save the mother and that indirectly kills the child is not unjust. The right to life can be compared to the right to private property. The right to property provides that one has a right to legitimately acquired property, but not a right to possess everything. Similarly the right to life gives a specific entitlement freedom from deliberately lethal commissions or omissions, and just because this is a difficult project does not mean that the right is nonexistent.

Thomson fails to see that there is an absolute character to the right to life, a right to be free from deliberate and intentional lethal actions performed by others when one is not guilty of acts of formal lethal aggression. The right to life demands that all refrain from deliberate and willful lethal commissions or omissions against innocent human life, and it demands that ordinary medical treatments be given to all persons.[73] It does not require that heroic acts of fortitude be taken in all cases to preserve and protect human life, even though it can require this in some instances.[74] And it does not demand that extraordinary medical treatments be given in all cases, even though there may not be anything objectionable with providing them in some instances. Clearly he does not because this would be formally categorized as an extraordinary medical treatment.

---

[72] *Ibid*. The only rights that others have to one's body are those given by the mother, thus a purely consensual theory of rights that is contrary to a theory of rights based on human nature.

[73] *Ibid*. P. 12. Thomson enunciates the terms of the right to life in part here by affirming the obligations of all individuals to refrain from intentional and deliberate lethal acts against others who are not material aggressors.

[74] For example, the right to life could demand that a national leader undergo radically painful surgery if it was certain that his death would cause the deaths of many innocent persons. The common good can require extraordinary measures to be taken for the well-being of an entire community, but these instances are admittedly rare.

The demands of the right to life remain the same throughout these changing circumstances, however, and they required that no deliberately lethal omissions or commissions be taken against innocent human life. What constitutes a lethal omission changes in different circumstances, but that does not invalidate the fundamental requirements of the right to life.

Thomson believes that Finnis improperly construes the nature of the right to life with his Hohfeldian rights analysis, but she fails to see that the right to life does give a Hohfeldian right to be free from deliberately lethal commissions or omissions. She is mystified by the fact that the right to life is defined as a right to a condition and not to an action. But she fails to see that the establishment of that condition makes certain forebearances and commissions incumbent on others, and in this way we see the Hohfeldian right generated. Thomson implies that the right to life is problematic because it is not clear that it gives a right to use other means to preserve life or the right to continue using any and all available means to support one's life.

The strength of the duties incumbent on others to protect innocent human life depends on the abilities of the persons involved to fulfill these duties. If one must use means that require the exercise of radical and heroic fortitude and which place one's own life in imminent danger, then the action could not be made an obligatory under justice. But if less than heroic actions were required to preserve life, life saving actions would then be demanded by justice. Thus, if one only had to throw a life ring to a drowning man, it would be a grave injustice not to do so. But if saving the man's life demanded that one jump into shark-infested waters, no violation of justice or obligation would be incurred by refraining from doing this.

2. Thomson does not deny the existence of a right to life, but only that this right includes an absolute requirement that the mother not withdraw support from the child.[75] She argues that having a right to life does not give one the right to use another's body without any restriction. It is true that the right to life does not give a right to invade another's body, but that does not mean that the other person can maim and dismember the child who has

---

[75] *Ibid.*

lodged within her body. What she fails to recall is that the unborn child has the right to life because of an action that was taken by the mother. Thomson makes the child's right to life out as if the mother had absolutely nothing to do with the unborn child living in the mother's womb. She makes it appear as if the child assaulted her and forced its way into the mother without the mother having had anything whatsoever to make that possible. She fails to see that the mother is not purely the victim of the child and does not affirm that in most cases the mother was the agent causing the child's existence.

Thomson has ignored the serious difficulty that her analysis cannot determine what constitutes an objectively unjust abortion. She argues that the right to life means we have a right not to be killed unjustly.[76] But the critical question is what constitutes an unjust killing. Abortions in the case of rape, or where the woman did not want to become pregnant would be just abortions for Thomson. But her theory implies that an unjust killing of an unborn child would be one where the child was killed even though it did not present an unacceptable burden to the mother. This would seem to be the only actual situation where an abortion would be unjust. The only other hypothetical situation where an abortion would be unjust in her theory would be where the mother had an abortion performed when she consented to the child's generation, but denied the child the right to use her body. But this situation is so irrational that it would seem that it is in fact impossible for abortion to be unjust for Thomson, for her principles allow a woman to rationalize any abortion by asserting that the child imposed too great a burden on her.

Traditional morality has been able to identify just and unjust abortions clearly and more persuasively than has Thomson. It has held that they are just when they are unintended consequences of therapeutic actions undertaken regrettably as the last and only reasonably means of saving the life of the mother. Abortive acts are unjust when they deliberately, freely, directly and with consent aim at destroying the child by either act or omission. Thomson cannot make a clear distinction such as this in her scheme. The classical tradition has considered abortion after rape unjust because the child

---

[76] *Ibid*. P. 13.

too is the victim of the rapist.[77] The woman has a right to defend herself against the rapist, but not against the child whose existence is also a consequence of the actions of the rapist and is not an aggressor against the woman as is the rapist.

Thomson's argument about the morality of abortion is also questionable because of her understanding of the moral malice of the act. In abortion, a positive choice is made to eliminate a being that is either fully human and personal, or is on an immediate trajectory toward the fully human and personal. In either case, the aim of the action, even though it may not be the aim of the agent, is to abolish a human life. In this, one sees the moral malice of abortion which is that it deliberately aims at the destruction of human life. A homicidal act is not immoral because it destroys personal life, but rather because human life is destroyed. As was shown in the previous chapter, the presumption should be in favor of assuming that unborn human life is personal, but even if it is not, the moral certainty remains that it is human life, and to deliberately seek to destroy innocent human life is immoral.

## CONCLUSION

In this chapter, I have sought to deal with the most forceful arguments for abortion that have been presented in the past decade and a half, and I have sought to show that there are profound deficiencies in their arguments. Neither have they persuasively argued for the permissibility of abortion. Abortion is in fact little more than deliberate killing of the defenseless innocent unborn to promote one's own convenience. If the case is to be made for the morality of direct abortion, it will have to come from arguments and reasons other than those presented by Thomson and Harrison. Neither have shown sufficient insight in to the nature of abortion to present arguments in defense of it, and they have not overcome the claim that abortion is immoral because it is the deliberate

---

[77] See: Grisez, Germain: *Abortion: The Myths, the Realities and the Arguments*, P. 168. Grisez points out that the Catholic tradition did not permit exceptions to its ban on direct abortion, even to save the life of the mother. The only noteworthy moral theologian who accepted rape as an indication for abortion was Thomas Sanchez in his *Disputationem de Sancto Matrimonio Sacramento* (Antwerp, 1616) ix, 20, 7-9, but this position was never endorsed by any official teaching.

destruction of innocent human life. Abortion is a highly problematic and troubling issue, and understanding its morality requires far more insight than have been provided by Harrison and Thomson.

# CHAPTER THREE
# INFANT CARE REVIEW COMMITTEES: THEIR MORAL RESPONSIBILITIES

The moral duties of infant care review committees (ICRCs) have become a widely discussed issue in recent years among physicians, ethicists and legal scholars. It now appears as if these committees will come to have a great deal of responsibility over the care and treatment of handicapped newborns, and it is becoming important to outline their moral duties in this role. Very broad formal and procedural guidelines for their proceedings have been suggested by other authors, but in this chapter I wish to present a fuller account of what is morally required of these committees. Ethics committees had their beginning in the decision rendered by the court in the Matter of *Karen Quinlan*.[1] In this decision, the court urged health care professionals, physicians and families to consult with ethics committees in difficult cases so that there could be full, free and open discussion of treatment issues. Generally, this proposal was not heeded by medical professionals or parents, largely because most seemed to want to preserve the traditional prerogatives reserved to them. As a result, few institutions established ethics committees after the *Quinlan* decision.[2] And in the years that followed this decision, only Catholic hospitals established ethics committees in large numbers.

Infant care review committees received their major impetus from the infamous Bloomington Baby Doe case for, in response to the death of the baby, the Department of Health and Human Services issued regulations to prevent the denial of care and medical treatment to handicapped children for the sole reason that they were handicapped.[3] These regulations were based on section 504 of the Rehabilitation Act of 1973 and these regulations stated that:

---

[1] Levine, Carol. "Questions and (Some Very Tentative") Answers About Hospital Ethics Committees", *Hastings Center Report*, June 1984. P. 9.

[2] Cranford, Ronald, E., and Doudera, Edward, A., "The Emergence of Institutional Ethics Committees", *Law, Medicine and Health Care*, Feb. 1984. P. 14.

[3] Levine. *op. cit.*, P. 10.

> No otherwise qualified handicapped individual. . . .shall, solely by reason of his handicap, be excluded from the participation in, be denied the benefits of, or be subjected to discrimination under any program or activity receiving federal financial assistance.[4]

Federal hotlines were initiated for the reporting of possible violations of this regulation, and many medical associations immediately protested these rules. Through a long series of negotiations, HHS accepted the legitimacy of infant care review committees when they were used in conjunction with federal hotlines.[5] The limited acceptance of these committees, along with the growing awareness that the traditional relationship between parents, patients and physicians was no longer adequate, spurred the present interest in infant care review committees. The Department of Health and Human Services did not view ICRCs as a substitute for the requirements of Section 504, but merely as an additional measure instituted to further protection for handicapped newborns and to promote quality medical decision-making.

Infant care review committees hold out a promise of significant benefits. They could make it less necessary for law enforcement agencies to intervene if they could guarantee that the rights of handicapped infants to normal care and ordinary medical treatments would not be violated. These committees could bring together some of the best minds in medicine, law and ethics to examine and resolve some critical problems in contemporary infant care.[6]

To study the moral responsibilities of infant care review committees, I shall begin by briefly surveying the various roles and functions suggested by leading authorities for these committees. Then I will examine some of the concerns and problems that have been expressed about ICRCs. Finally, the general and specific moral

---

[4] See: Richard McCormick, S.J. *Health and Medicine in the Catholic Tradition*, (New York: Crossroads Books, 1984) P. 146.

[5] Levine, *op. cit.* P. 9.

[6] See: Department of Health and Human Services, *Infant Care Review Committee Interim Model Guidelines*, 45 CFR 1340 Section IV A, Basic Functions.

obligations of these to handicapped infants, parents, physicians and society will be studied.

# A
# INFANT CARE REVIEW COMMITTEES: THEIR ROLE AND FUNCTIONS

The three general functions of infant care review committees will be examined here. Virtually all authorities and commentators agree that ICRCs can serve a general educational function for both health care facility staff members and the public at large. They also agree that those committees can review treatment proposals both prospectively and retrospectively. And ICRCs are also seen as agencies which can assist in the formation of guidelines, standards and norms for the care of handicapped infants.

## 1
## The Educational Function of Infant Care Review Committees

While there is general agreement that ICRCs should educate health care facility staff members and the public at large concerning the care and treatment of handicapped infants, there is no unity on what should be taught by these committees. The American Academy of Pediatrics asserted that these committees should educate parents about the means of treatment available in health care facilities and in the community for handicapped children.[7] However, these tasks seem to be better suited to other bodies, and most authorities agree that ICRCs should limit themselves to instruction in ethical matters. The most common view is that infant care review committees should inform parents, physicians and health care staff members of their ethical responsibilities.

There is some debate as to whether ethics committees should merely provide a forum for discussion of ethical issues, or whether they should assume an explicitly pedagogical role in which they

---

[7] American Academy of Pediatrics, "Guidelines for Infant Bioethics Committees" (Unpublished manuscript), section VII, A, "Educational Functions". P. 6.

would teach determinate ethical principles and rules.[8] One leading authority has asserted that ICRCs should link societal values with developments in institutions, but it is not clear what this means.[9] In contrast, some ethics committees in Catholic institutions have assumed a wider role and have aimed at teaching about the social implications of certain medical practices and policies, but his function has not been widely regarded as necessary for infant care review committees.[10]

## 2
## Infant Care Review Committees and Case Review

Almost all authorities agree that ICRCs have a role in reviewing the treatment given to or proposed for handicapped infants.[11] A number of writers have asserted that infant care review committees should not make decisions about the cases they review, but they are not clear in what they say about this.[12] If this assertion means that ICRCs should not make medical decisions about treatments given to or proposed for handicapped infants, then no objections could be raised.[13] It would seem that ICRCs, by their very nature, are to aim at coming to moral judgments about actions

---

[8] Levine, *op. cit.* P. 10.

[9] Cranford and Doudera. *Op. cit.* P. 14.

[10] Kelly, S. Margaret, John, DC, Ph.D. and McCarthy, Donald, G. *Ethics Committees: A Challenge for Catholic Health Care* (St. Louis: Catholic Health Association, 1984) P. 5.

[11] Cranford and Doudera. *Op. cit.* Pp. 16, 17. Also see: Alan R. Fleishcman and Thomas H. Murray, "Ethics Committees for Infants Doe?" *Hastings Center Report*, Dec. 1983. Pp. 8, 9; and American Academy of Pediatrics, *Guidelines*. *Op. cit.* P. 3.

[12] Cranford and Doudera, *op. cit.* P. 17. Benjamin Freedman, "One Philosopher's Experience on an Ethics Committee", *Hastings Center Report*, April 1981. Pp. 20-21.

[13] It would be hard to consider ethics committees to be truly such if they were either explicitly or implicitly forbidden to make ethical judgments as it would be impossible to consider prognosis committees medical committees if they were forbidden to make medical judgments.

or treatment proposals, but to deny them the freedom to do this would be to defeat their primary purpose. That ICRCs should make ethical judgments does not mean that they should replace the traditional *loci* of medical decision-making, but it does imply that these traditional forms of medical decision-making should be subjected to strict ethical scrutiny and that all decision-makers should be held accountable for any irresponsible actions.

Most authorities do not object to infant care review committees making ethical judgments about treatments or proposals for treatment. But at the far end of the spectrum, one author suggest that ICRCs should only decide who should decide about the provision of treatment.[14] It is difficult to take this suggestion seriously, however, for shortly after making it, the author asserted that the parents should make decisions about the treatment of children unless they were judged incompetent by a court.[15] This view would unduly restrict the freedom of action of ICRCs and it is one that has not been shared by many authors.

Case review can either be prospective or retrospective. In prospective review of cases, it has been argued that committees should obtain all of the relevant facts of the case, identify the important issues, resolve the differences between parents and physicians, affirm the complexity or difficulty of the cases and recommend intervention of law enforcement agencies if necessary.[16] A serious problem almost all writers mention with the prospective review of cases is that of determining when ICRCs should intervene prospectively. Some have said that infant care review committees should intervene whenever life-sustaining treatments are proposed for withdrawal.[17] Others have suggested that they only intervene when requested to do so by physicians, parents, or staff members.[18]

---

[14] Fleischman and Murray, *op. cit.* P. 9.

[15] *Ibid*.

[16] *Ibid*.

[17] American Academy of Pediatrics, "Guidelines", . VII, C. 2, P. 7.

[18] Freedman, *op. cit.* P. 20.

Another difficult problem mentioned by some authors is that of determining the authority of judgments or recommendations made by infant care review committees. Some claim that ICRCs recommendations or resolutions be binding on those who treat handicapped infants, while others would hold that they should be binding on them in varying degrees according to the circumstances.[19] When committees do intervene prospectively, there is little agreement among authorities as to how they should evaluate treatment proposals. Some assert that ICRCs should only require that "reasonable" or "appropriate" actions be taken in behalf of handicapped infants, or that of the "best interests" of the child be promoted.[20] Others have asserted that the dignity of the parents and physicians should be affirmed and promoted by ICRCs. But to my knowledge, few notable authors recommend that institutional ethics committees intervene when the *rights* of the infant are in jeopardy. The absence of an affirmation of this should be of concern, for it was in such a situation that the Baby Doe regulations were specifically promulgated.

In their prospective review of cases, some writers have suggested that ICRCs should not aim at reaching a consensus in their judgments, but should merely settle for a wide-ranging discussion of the issues.[21] And virtually all authorities agree that courts and law enforcement agencies should only be allowed to intervene and investigate as a matter of last resort.[22]

### 3
### Policy and Guideline Formation

Most authorities hold that infant care review committees should have a role in the formation of policies and guidelines for the

---

[19] Levine, *op. cit.* P. 11.

[20] See: Fleischman and Murray, *op. cit.* p. 9; Levine, *op. cit.* P. 10; and American Academy of Pediatrics, "Guidelines" *op. cit.* VII, C. 7, P. 9.

[21] *Ibid.* VII, C, 6, P. 9.

[22] Cranford and Doudera, *op. cit.* p. 19; Fleischman and Murray. *op. cit.* Pp. 7, 8.

treatment of handicapped infants, but there is not much agreement on the nature of these guidelines.[23] No writers have suggested that guidelines contrary to institutional bylaws be adopted or endorsed by infant care review committees. Being predominantly procedural and formal, the guidelines which have been thus far proposed have not demonstrated that they could effectively protect her rights of handicapped infants in critical situations.[24] As there is little or no mention of these guidelines in Section 504 of the Rehabilitation Act, one can readily draw the conclusion that the primary objective of these guidelines is the protection of parents and physicians. Most authors claim that they wish to promote high quality medical decision making, but they are not specific concerning the nature of this improved decision making.

If any judgments concerning their moral responsibilities of ICRCs are to be made, it would be to not only necessary to understand their roles and functions, but to also grasp the problems and concerns which surround ICRCs. The aim of this next section will be to examine some of these problems and concerns before studying the moral obligations of these committees.

## B
### INFANT CARE REVIEW COMMITTEES: CONCERNS AND PROBLEMS

There are five general areas of concern with infant care review committees:

1). Probably the most significant concern with ICRCs is that they could really become dominated by the interests of one or a small number of groups or individuals to the detriment of

---

[23] American Academy of Pediatrics, "Guidelines." *op. cit.* P. 3; Levine, *op. cit.*, P. 10; and Cranford and Doudera. *op. cit.* P. 16.

[24] See: American Academy of Pediatrics, "A Proposal for an Ethics Committee", *Hastings Center Report*, Dec. 1983. Pp. 6, 7.

physicians, patients, and handicapped infants.[25] Many committees not only restrict admission to the committees themselves, but also to the proceedings of the committees.[26] Limiting access to the committees can be seen as a way of overcoming resistance to them in hospitals.[27] Most committees limit the access of nurses to committees, and a 1982 survey found that only 31 per-cent of committees allowed them to present cases, and only 50 per-cent allowed them to attend meetings.[28] Access to the proceedings of the committees is often limited in order to protect members from civil suit.[29] It has been suggested by one authority that committees be used as a public relations tool to justify "unpopular" decisions to discontinue unpopular services.[30]

[25] Levine. *op. cit.* P. 11; Cranford and Doudera. *op. cit.* Pp. 17, 18. These committees can be readily abused to protect those who wish to eliminate handicapped infants, for they can be employed to mitigate responsibility for difficult decisions. In 1964, Dr. R. F. Tredgold published an article in *Lancet* noting the difficulties that physicians had in deciding to perform abortions. "See his: "Psychiatric Indications for Termination of Pregnancy." P. 2, (1964) 1253. In response to this article, many physicians wrote urging the formation of these committees. One psychiatrist said: "[B]ut since the decision is so harrowing and the individual psychiatrist is so influenced by prejudice, conscious or unconscious, surely it would be wise to share this grave responsibility with colleagues and with, perhaps, a non-professional woman of common sense and childbearing age." M. P. Joyston-Bechal, "Letter", *Lancet*, P. 1 (1965), P. 318. ICRCs as well as other medical ethics committees can be put to the same unethical use, but it would be regrettable to do so.

[26] See: Lo, M.D., Bernard. "Behind Closed Door: Promises and Pitfalls of Ethics Committees", *The New England Journal of Medicine*, July 2, 1987. P. 47.

[27] *Ibid.*

[28] See: Youngner, S; Jackson, D. L; Coulton, C; Junkialis, B; Smith, E; " A Survey of Hospital Ethics Committees", *Critical Care Medicine*, 1983, Vol, 11. Pp. 905-6.

[29] Winslow, G, "From Loyalty to Advocacy: A New Metaphor for Nursing" *Hastings Center Report*, 1984, Vol. 14, No. 3, Pp. 32-40. Also see: Cranford, R; Hester, F.A; Ashley, B. Z. "Institutional Ethics Committees: Issues of Confidentiality and Immunity", *Law, Medicine and Health Care*, 1985, Vol. 13. Pp. 52-60.

[30] Summers, J. W., "Closing Unprofitable Services: Ethical Issues and Management Responses", *Hospital Health Service Administration*, 1985, Vol. 30. Pp. 8-28.

Reports have shown that it is relatively easy for physicians to dominate these groups and use them to promote their own private interests.[31] This problem has been less acute with ethics committees in Catholic health care facilities, as they have generally had greater diversity in their composition and membership.[32] Virtually all authorities assert that infant care review committees should strive to attain diverse membership and thereby limit the harmful effects of domination by a single group or individual.

2). Holding infant care review committees accountable for their actions is another major area of concern.[33] ICRCs often fail to provide the safeguards that court proceedings do, for they often do not provide for an equivalent to guardians *ad litem* and they often do not write their decision down on medical records for fear that their decisions could be "discoverable", thereby exposing their members to civil suit.[34]

ICRCs appear to have a problems similar to that which Institutional Review Boards (IRBs) had when they first began. IRBs often failed to adequately protect the rights of research subjects against unethical research, and it is thus feared by some that ICRCs could jeopardize the rights of handicapped infants by being neglectful of their duties to argue in behalf of their rights.[35] ICRCs appear vulnerable to this possibility, and most authors call for measures to make ICRCs accountable for their judgments and actions. Ethics committees are often pressured to reach agreement on cases that can often be ethically questionable even though agreement or

---

[31] President's Commission for the Study of Ethical Problems in Medicine and Biomedical and Behavioral Research, *Deciding to Forego Life-Sustaining Treatment* (Washington: U. S. Government Printing Office, 1983) P. 446.

[32] Levine, *op. cit.* P. 12.

[33] Fleischman and Murray, *op. cit.* P. 9.

[34] Levine, *op. cit.* P. 11; Fleischman and Murray, *op. cit.* P. 9.

[35] Lo, Bernard. "Behind Closed Doors: Promises and Pitfalls of Ethics Committees". P. 48.

consensus does not mean ethical infallibility.[36] The need to reach consensus or group decisions can even impair ethical decision making as committee members can be pressured to reach certain decisions or avoid controversial issues.[37] Ethics committees can fall into "groupthink" where consensus is reached too easily. Ethics committees are not immune to making decisions on unsubstantiated or uncorroborated evidence. Without adequate safeguards, it is quite possible that ICRCs could become culpable cooperators in unjust actions against handicapped infants.

3). A further problem with these committees is that their roles and functions appear to be so vaguely defined that they could readily abrogate to themselves the roles of parents, physicians, surrogate decision-makers, health care institutions, law enforcement agencies or the courts. Ethics committees sometimes function without goals. One committee claimed, "We have never formally stated in writing the exact purpose or purposes of our committee but have decided to proceed in an informal manner. . . We felt that to formalize our objectives might be counterproductive to the work of our committee."[38] The absence of precise objectives is a serious issue because it is not certain that ICRCs have the competence or authority to assume any of these roles completely. Related to this concern is that of the possible violations of the rights of privacy and confidentiality of interested parties by ICRCs because of inadequate procedural standards and regulations. To counter this possibility, some authors have strongly urged forceful measures to protect the

[36] Janis, I. L.; Mann, L. *Decision-making: A Psychological Analysis of Conflict, Choice and Commitment.* (New York: Free Press, 1977). Also see: George, A. "Toward A More Soundly Based Foreign Policy." in *Commission on the Organization of the Government for the Conduct of Foreign Policy*, Appendix B. (Washington, D.C: Government Printing Office, 1975.)

[37] Kushner, T; Gibson, J. M; "Institutional Ethics Committees Speak for Themselves" in Cranford, R. E; Doudera, A. E., eds. *op. cit.* Pp. 96-105.

[38] American Academy of Pediatrics, "Guidelines", *op. cit.*, VIII, P. 11; Levine, *op. cit.* p. 12; Department of Health and Human Services. *op. cit.* B 3, P. 7.

privacy and confidentiality of all involved parties.[39]

4). There have been few reported instances of infant care review committees requiring excessive treatment, and it is quite possible that these committees might become biased in favor of unjustifiable non-treatment or undertreatment. A number of authors have urged that the activities of ICRCs be severely limited, and if these proposals are accepted, the power of these committees to require treatment could become severely restricted.[40] This problem could be minimized if there were more specific and concrete guidelines of ICRCs, for the guidelines being proposed today for most committees have little capability for compelling committees to require ethically demanded and justified treatment.

5). Up to the present time, practically all the procedures and guidelines suggested for ICRCs have been purely procedural and formal. This raises the possibility that ICRCs could intervene without justification, or fail to intervene, in review cases when such intervention would be justified or morally required. Enactment of sound, concise, precise and substantive norms and standards seems therefore to be necessary for ICRCs.

In light of these issues and concerns about the roles and functions of infant care review committees, it is now possible to discuss their general and specific moral responsibilities. While this discussion of their responsibilities will focus primarily on their moral obligations, some attention will be given to their legal obligations to the extent that they bear on their moral duties and responsibilities.

## C
## THE MORAL RESPONSIBILITIES
## OF INFANT CARE REVIEW COMMITTEES

---

[39] Fleischman and Murray, *op. cit.* p. 9. They would wish to remove all serious ethical debate about the morality of acts and treatment proposals and only discuss the issue of who is to decide the issue of providing treatment. The net effect of this would be to radically limit the activities of these committees.

[40] May, William, E. *Human Existence, Medicine and Ethics*, (Chicago: Franciscan Herald Press, 1977), p. 26. Also see John Simon, Charles Powers and Jon Gunnemann, *The Ethical Investigator* (New Haven: Yale University Press, 1972) Pp. 22-25.

Before discussing the general moral duties of these committees, it is necessary to state that those who establish ICRCs have a strict moral duty and obligation to structure them so that they can fulfill their duties in full freedom. If ICRCs are so restricted in their actions and authority that they cannot execute what is morally required of them, then any attempt to impose moral responsibilities on them would be futile.

Infant care review committees have four moral responsibilities in all of their functions and roles.

1). All ICRCs are bound by the duties imposed on them by what has come to be known as the Kew Gardens Principle. This principle asserts that all moral agents are required to take actions which do not entail grave risk for them if those actions would prevent another from loosing a fundamental human good or from experiencing grave suffering.[41] For infant care review committees, this principle means that they must take whatever actions are reasonably within their means to prevent handicapped infants from suffering grave harm or injury by willful commissions or omissions performed by other moral agents.

2). All infant review committees are under a common and ordinary moral obligation to protect innocent human life from direct and deliberate lethal commissions or omissions.[42] This principle is correlative to the Kew Gardens Principle, but it affirms the nature of this obligation in a more precise and technical manner.

3). In all of their actions concerning the protection of handicapped newborns, infant care review committees are morally required to adopt the morally safer course of action.[43] This does not mean that ICRCs must adopt the safest course of action in all circumstances, but only that they must act to guarantee that handicapped infants not be denied any reasonable chance for life and improved health. This principle does not endorse moral rigorism, for it promotes and encourages moral responsibility, responsibility,

---

[41] McHugh, John, O.P., and Callan, Charles, O.P., *Moral Theology: A Complete Course*. (New York: Wagner, 1929) Vol. II, Pp. 112, 113; Vol. I. Pp. 15-17.

[42] *Ibid*. Vol. I. P. 268.

[43] Department of Health and Human Services, *Child Abuse Treatment Act*. P. 15.

prudence and respect for fragile and innocent human life.

4). All infant care review committees are morally obliged to promote, endorse and support laws and efforts of law enforcement agencies which seek to responsibly protect the moral rights of handicapped infants to ordinary medical treatments and care.[44] ICRCs are not meddlesome "do-gooders", exceeding their authority when they do this, but are only fulfilling a common and ordinary jurisprudential duty incumbent on all moral agents.[45] Because the law is more precise and specific than are moral principles, norms and rules, it is better able to protect the rights of all parties, there is a moral duty to support it when it is administered responsibly. By doing this, infant care review committees are better able to fulfill their moral responsibilities toward handicapped infants.

These are the general moral duties of infant care review committees, but there are also some specific moral responsibilities incumbent on these committees that must be mentioned.

## 1
## The Moral Duties of Infant Care Review Committees In Education and Case Review

In all of their case review activities, infant care review committees are to gather all possible relevant factual data concerning the cases in question. All aspects of their reviews and investigations are to be properly and accurately documented and recorded to protect all parties involved.

When infant care review committees function in their educative role, they are to recall that their primary function is to instruct physicians, staff members and parents of their moral duties. ICRCs are not simply to provide forums for discussion, or aim at replacing legitimate regulatory functions of government.[46] ICRCs

---

[44] Freedman, *op. cit.* P. 21.

[45] Cranford and Doudera, *op. cit.* P. 15.

[46] American Academy of Pediatrics, "Guidelines". *op. cit.* VII, C, 2, p. 7; Department of Health and Human Services, *Interim Guidelines, op. cit.* VI, A.1, P. 13.

are to take a pedagogical role in their educational activities because this is required by the principle that the safer course of action is to be followed. Infant care review committees are to train health care professionals in their moral duties toward handicapped infants. They are to give precise ethical guidance which, above all else, is to positively promote the rights of handicapped infants, especially in complex and difficult cases. In this role, they are to instruct in the requirements of ordinary moral duties and in what is demanded by the safer course of action in various circumstances. And it is also a moral obligation for these committees to instruct parents and physicians in their moral obligations toward the law.

In their roles of retrospective and prospective case review, infant care review committees might not be required to make medical decisions, but that should not prohibit them from making ethical judgments about treatments or treatment proposals. To prohibit them from making these judgments is morally equivalent to prohibiting physicians from making ethical judgments concerning clinical cases brought to their attention.

In both prospective and retrospective case review, ICRCs are to take the safer course of moral action and intervene to review three separate kinds of cases. First, they are to intervene as a matter of moral obligation and make ethical judgments in cases where life sustaining treatments are being proposed for withdrawal such that the infant might suffer grave harm or death from the withdrawal.[47] This is required because there is imminent danger that the withdrawal of such treatments or care could be directly lethal or would be a violation of the rights of the infant to care and obligatory medical treatment.

Second, infant care review committees are morally required to intervene in cases where possibly medically beneficial care or treatments is being proposed for withdrawal or have actually been denied a handicapped infant. This is morally required because it is quite possible that grave harm could come to the infant if such proposals were carried out, and therefore, taking the safer course of action would require review.

---

[47] This is required for the reason that there are so few, if any, situations in which nutrition and fluids could be legitimately withdrawn from infants that the strong possibility that any denial of nutrition and fluids would be an instance of culpably direct killing.

Third, infant care review committees are required to review cases where nutrition and fluids are being proposed for withdrawal or have actually been removed.[48] Taking the safer course of action requires this because there are few, if any, situations in which definitive denial of food and/or fluids would not be direct killing. Whenever nutrition and hydration are of nutritional and hydrational value and can be ingested and metabolized by the individual without severe pain and can be provided, they should be given by health care personnel.

Nutrition and fluids are not medical treatments, but are basic resources of the body whose provision sustains life and whose withdrawal certainly causes death.[49] Their provision directly supports the natural functions of the body and its natural defenses against diseases. Because they are not specifically medical treatments, their provision should be regulated by principles other than those which govern the administration of medical treatments. Nutrition and fluids are aspects of normal care and should be given whenever they can meet the nutritional and hydrational needs of the patient, as they are of benefit to the patient when they do this. There is nothing immoral whatsoever about feeding an individual if this will sustain life, and there very well might be something seriously immoral in denying nutrition and fluids to a patient so that death is brought about by this denial. Taking the safer course of action requires that one avoid the risk of unjust killing by providing food and water when they can preserve life. Food and fluids are different from medical treatments because they are not directly therapeutic as they do not directly and proximately correct or ameliorate clinically diagnosable conditions. If anything constitutes medical abandonment, it is the refusal to provide food and fluids to persons whose lives can be sustained by them. The Vatican recognized this in its *Declaration on Euthanasia* when it asserted that normal care was to be given to all patients, even to

---

[48] Dennis J. Horan and Edward Grant, "The Legal Aspects of Withdrawing Nourishment", *Journal of Legal Medicine*, Vol. 5, No. 4 (1985) Pp. 618-619.

[49] Sacred Congregation for the Doctrine of the Faith, *Declaration on Euthanasia*, sec. IV.

those who were terminally ill.[50]

In both prospective and retrospective case review, infant care review committees are to uphold the requirements of the law. This requirement specifically implies that infant care review committees are not to be used in any fashion that might impede the enforcement of the law seeking to protect the rights of handicapped infants. They are to instruct individuals in their duty to report suspected cases of child abuse and neglect, and they are to reprimand individuals or organizations which fail to do this.[51] ICRCs are not only to report cases of child abuse when they judge that there is sufficient evidence for a conviction, but even when there is only a suspicion that neglect or abuse is occurring. And in both retrospective and prospective case review, infant care review committees are to take steps to assure that their actions are carried out.

Infant care review committees also have specific moral duties in their role of assisting in the development of policies and guidelines, and these will be examined in the next part.

## 2
## Moral Duties in Policy and Guideline Development

The fundamental duty of ICRCs in the development of policies, guidelines, norms and standards is to assure that these are not merely procedural, formal and subjective, but substantive, concrete and specific. This is required by the principle of the safer course of action, as failure to demand this places handicapped infants in imminent danger. Guidelines cannot aim at merely being "feasible", for these would not guarantee the rights of infants to morally obligatory medical treatments in complex and difficult situations. Guidelines cannot aim at being merely being "reasonable", "appropriate" or in the "best interests" of the child either, for these are so formal that they will not assure protection

---

[50] Department of Health and Human Services, *Child Abuse Treatment Act*. P. 16.

[51] "Task Force on Supportive Care, Supportive Care Plan: Its Meaning and Application" (Unpublished Manuscript) Oct. 1983. P. 1.

of the rights of the child to normal care and ordinary medical treatments. Most of the criteria currently being proposed are purely procedural and formal, and by themselves they cannot impose any specific concrete and practical moral duties on anyone. Most norms and standards regulating the activities of infant care review committees must concretely aim at protecting the rights of handicapped to morally required medical treatments.

Norms and standards endorsed or promoted by ICRCs must be in compliance with civil and criminal laws protecting the rights of handicapped infants against discriminatory acts. There is an implicit requirement in this demand which forbids ICRCs from endorsing policies and guidelines which violate the moral rights of physicians, health care institutions and parents. And it is particularly important that ICRCs endorse policies which protect the privacy and confidentiality of all individuals and parties involved in the treatment of handicapped newborns.

Recently it has been suggested that some handicapped infants be included in a treatment category called "supportive care only", in which no life-sustaining measures or treatments would be provided.[52] Policies such as these, when suggested for handicapped newborns who are not imminently and unavoidably dying and for whom nutrition and fluids and other medical treatments would be of benefit are objectionable. There are instances in which palliative care could be provided morally because nutrition and fluids could not be ingested, but a policy of permitting infants who are not imminently and unavoidably dying is immoral.

It has been suggested by some authorities that "nontreatment" as a medical policy is morally legitimate when various kinds of other treatments would be of clear benefit to a child and when "nontreatment" would do nothing to improve the child's

---

[52] Weir, Robert. *Selective Nontreatment of Handicapped Newborns.* (New York: Oxford University Press, 1984) P. 216. Weir claims that there are many meanings of "nontreatment" but in only one of them will an infant not die imminently from the denial of treatment. His views of the nature of "nontreatment" are so elastic, however, that he considers the administration of potassium injections to infants who will not die when all other treatments are removed to be a form of "nontreatment".

clinical picture.[53] Adopting "nontreatment" as an option is not morally tolerable when readily available treatments and food and water would sustain the infant's life is nothing but a violation of the rights of the child by omission.

There are quite a number of specific clinical conditions from which infants can suffer and in the final section the moral responsibilities of ICRCs to infants with some of these specific conditions will be considered.

## 3
## Moral Responsibilities of ICRCs in Special Cases

It has been suggested by some authors that compassionate and humane treatment of infants with various conditions such as Lesch-Nyhan disease, Tay-Sachs disease, hydroencephaly, trisomy 13 and other ailments should be withdrawn or withheld.[54] The justification for this position is that the suffering experienced by the children with these conditions is so severe that death would be preferable to life. This position is highly objectionable, however, because it is implied that nutrition and fluids would also be removed so that the children would be starved or dehydrated to death. As a result, these children are not allowed to die, but are rather killed by culpable omission. Denying that food and water would not do anything to improve their condition and it would introduce a certainly lethal cause which did not previously exist. Removal of nutrition and fluids does not cause the child to die due to a condition from which he or she is suffering, but rather it introduces a new and independent cause of death.

It has been suggested that it would be morally permissible to bring certain handicapped newborns to death by directly killing

---

[53] *Ibid*. P. 235. It also seems that he considers these children to be candidates for direct killing, for many of them will not die imminently when all other treatments are withdrawn, and therefore they can be directly killed by swift and painless injections.

[54] *Ibid*. P. 216. Weir argues that direct killing is morally tolerable when nothing can be done to prevent the suffering of an infant. It might even be mandatory to give lethal injections, according to Weir, to abide by the principle of nonfeasance.

them.[55] If it was judged that continued life was not in the best interests of the child, if the child suffered in the absence of treatment, and if death could be brought about painlessly, then it would not be immoral to directly kill a child, probably by lethal injection, in the opinion of some.[56] This is also quite objectionable because direct killing is never morally permissible, even when its motives are compassion and concern. Life is a basic and fundamental good and it can never become a burden to one in and of itself. The conditions from which one can suffer can become burdensome, but life itself cannot become burdensome. Giving lethal injections to infants makes physicians killers and it violates the medical canon "do no harm". Death is never a friend of a child, and while it is not an absolute evil, it is never something which should be deliberately and directly chosen. The moral absolute against direct killing should be compared to the moral absolute against rape. While rape might bring some psychological benefits to the rapist, it is always wrong. Similarly, while directly lethal attacks on handicapped infants might some benefits to others, it is not something that should ever be chosen. Handicapped infants have an ordinary moral right not to be starved and dehydrated to death and they have an ordinary moral right not to be directly killed because someone thinks they are suffering too much.

When considering treatments to be given to spina bifida children, any and all readily available treatments which improve the clinical picture of the child should be given. Any treatment which palliates, alleviates or corrects their clinical conditions without undue burden to the parents or health care providers should be given as a matter of moral duty. Aggressive treatment of children with spina bifida should never be regarded as imposing harm on them, for example, when there is a prognosis that such treatments would improve the clinical condition of the child. But where a child with spina bifida has a prognosis of imminent death, aggressive treatment which cannot ward off death is useless and not obligatory. Even in this circumstance, palliative care and nutrition and fluids

---

[55] *Ibid.* P. 249.

[56] President's Commission, *op. cit.* P. 446.

should be given if possible so as to prevent the child from succumbing to the lack of these.

Infant care review committees should thus work to assure that infants with these conditions are not denied the care and medical treatments that are due them in these circumstances. "Do not resuscitate" orders should only be given for those handicapped infants who suffer from terminal illnesses and who are imminently and unavoidably dying. These orders should not be based on "quality of life" judgments, or on other standards such as the "benefit or burden" of resuscitation. Rather these orders should only be issued when it is clear that they cannot stave off death any longer.

## Conclusion

For all of the discussion of the responsibilities of infant care review committees in recent years, it appears that such committees have been badly underutilized in the recent past. One study showed that hospital ethics committees were only used once a year on the average in those hospitals which had instituted them. At the present time, there is a concerted effort to create a network of infant care review committees, and this effort should be viewed cautiously. Many authorities admit that there are not experienced ethicists to be found on most committees, and this could lead to highly objectionable practices and judgments by these committees. It is quite possible that ICRCs could be used in the future as shields against legitimate intervention by law enforcement agencies seeking to protect handicapped infants from abuse and neglect, and this would be unfortunate if it were to happen. Thus, it is imperative that ICRCs adopt strict moral standards and that they be closely monitored during their creation and growth. The existence and development of these institutions is desirable only if they enhance the protection of handicapped and aid in enforcing laws designed to protect them. They must not be allowed to become impediments to the enforcement of laws and regulations designed to protect handicapped infants, and they must be watched closely to assure that they achieve this end.

# SECTION TWO
# EUTHANASIA
# CHAPTER FOUR
# THE BROADENING SCOPE OF EUTHANASIA

Between 1986 and 1988, significant legal, social and ethical barriers to euthanasia were challenged and collapsed. Passive mercy killing by omission of beneficial and readily available forms of medical treatment and food and water from patients, either with or without their consent were given varying levels of legal and social acceptance. Because of this, our nation now stands on the brink of legalized mercy killing by lethal injection.

This view was confirmed in an article entitled "Court Paves Way to Remove Artificial Feeding" in the *American Medical News* which said the following about 1986:

> It was a watershed year for the ultimate issue in the so-called "right to die" area of medical ethics.
>
> The issue is whether it is ethical and legal for physicians after consultation with the families or parents of patients for whom there is no hope of recovery, to remove artificial feeding. The courts and the medical profession in 1986 seemed to make it clear that the actions are both ethical and legal--a bold step in an area of social policy that evolved quickly and decisively in just three short years.[1]

This chapter will attempt to give an account of the development of the mercy killing movement in this country in recent months by summarizing the findings of recent court cases and writings of exponents of the right to die.

## A
## MEDICO-LEGAL DEVELOPMENTS PROMOTING EUTHANASIA

---

[1] *American Medical News*, "Court Paves Way to Remove Artificial Feeding", by Mark Rust. January 2, 1987. P. 1.

# 1
## The Clarence Herbert Case

The case which introduced the contemporary mercy killing movement to this country was the case of Clarence Herbert. In August, 1982, Mr. Herbert, a race track guard in Los Angeles was admitted to Kaiser Permanente Hospital near Los Angeles for elective surgery to close an opening in his intestines. The operation was successful, but in the recovery room Mr. Herbert suffered respiratory distress followed by respiratory-cardiac arrest.[2] At the time of the arrest, the recovery room was not sufficiently staffed, and before he was revived he suffered severe anoxia with resultant brain damage.[3] He was placed on a respirator and given fluids by an intravenous line. From that point on, it was not fully clear what transpired, and the following facts must be gleaned from other sources, especially from testimony presented at the preliminary hearing.[4]

On August 28, two days after he experienced this trauma, Drs. Neil Barber and Robert Nejdl approached Mr. Herbert's wife Patsy for permission to remove the respirator.[5] According to Mrs. Herbert, the physicians told her that Mr. Herbert was "brain dead", which was not true, and they wanted her consent to remove the respirator.[6] Mrs. Herbert gathered her family together and they executed a written statement asserting that all life-support machines

---

[2] B. Steinbock, "The Removal of Mr. Herbert's Feeding Tube," *The Hastings Center Report*, Oct., 1983, P. 13.

[3] "Death Case Malpractice Discounted," *The Los Angeles Times*, Feb., 12, 1983, P. 30, Col. 2.

[4] See: D. Horan; and E. Grant. "The Legal Aspects of Withdrawing Nourishment", *The Journal of Legal Medicine*, 5, 4, 1984, P. 604. (Hereinafter referred to as *Legal Aspects*.)

[5] *Barber v. People*, 147 Cal. App. 3d 1006 Cal. Rptr. 484 (1983) P. 486.

[6] "Nurses Sparked Patient Death Probe", *Los Angeles Times*, Sept., 15, 1982, Section II, P. 4, col. I.

were to be removed from Mr. Herbert.[7] Drs. Barber and Nejdl carried out the family's wish despite the fact that Mr. Herbert had designated his sister-in-law to make decisions in event of his incompetency.[8] Despite the removal of the respirator, Mr. Herbert continued to breathe, and on August 30, Drs. Barber and Nejdl again approached the family and reportedly suggested that all life-support measures, including food and fluids, be removed.[9] But Mrs. Herbert later claimed that she could not recall if they specifically requested that food and water be removed.[10] However, on that day all hydrational support was withdrawn and Mr. Herbert expired on September 6, probably as a result of dehydration even though the death certificate listed diffuse encephalomalacia, secondary to anoxia, as the cause of death.[11]

A neurologist examined Mr. Herbert and determined that he had a "poor" prognosis for neurological recovery which remained current in his record until two days before his death and for four days after he was denied hydrational support.[12] This prognosis was by no means certain or precise, but it did indicate that Mr. Herbert's stupor was not necessarily irreversible. It appears as if the diagnosis and prognosis of the neurologist were ignored by Drs. Barber and Nejdl, and it is not clear why they were in such haste to remove his respirator and intravenous line, as standard medical practice would have dictated continuing respiratory and intravenous support for at least thirty days. There is a significant statistical difference between a "poor" prognosis for neurological recovery and a "hopeless" prognosis. Also, Mr. Herbert was neither "brain dead"

---

[7] Steinbock, *supra*, note 29, P. 13.

[8] "Nurse Sparked Patient Death Probe," P. 4, Col, I.

[9] Steinbock, *supra*, note 29, P. 13.

[10] *Ibid.*

[11] 195 Cal. Rptr. P. 487.

[12] Horan and Grant, *Legal Aspects*, P. 608.

nor imminently dying.[13]

The Los Angeles County District Attorney's office was required to investigate Mr. Herbert's death, and it issued a criminal complaint for murder against Drs. Barber and Nejdl. A pretrial hearing was marked by extensive testimony from a prominent medical ethicist supporting the contention that removal of food and fluids from Mr. Herbert was ethically sound.[14] The magistrate concluded that the complaint should be dismissed for three reasons: (1) the physicians did not "kill" Herbert, since the proximate cause of death was not their conduct but the diffuse encephalomalacia; (2) the physicians' conduct was not unlawful but in "good faith and sound ethical, medical judgment; and (3) the physicians' state of mind did not amount to malice."[15]

The California Second District Court of Appeals decided that the controlling legal principle was not the law against homicide, but the physicians' duty to act.[16] This court held that the cessation of "heroic" life support measures was to be viewed as an omission and not as an affirmative act.[17]

The court reasoned that every drop of intravenous fluids was comparable to a manually administered injection of medicine and could be withheld just as could manually administered medications or injections.[18] In making this judgment, the court turned its back on the most controversial aspect of this case and simply asserted that nutrition and hydration were fundamentally indistinguishable from other medical treatments. By refusing to consider the possibility that nutrition and fluids were to be provided according to principles other than those governing the administration of medical

---

[13] The neurologist never made such a diagnosis, and the prognosis of "poor" or "nil" could only have been made if he still retained some neurological functioning.

[14] Horan and Grant, *Legal Aspects*, P. 605.

[15] Steinbock, *supra*, note 29, Pp. 13-14.

[16] 195 Cal. Rptr. P. 490.

[17] *Ibid*. P. 490.

[18] *Ibid*.

treatments, it avoided the question of whether withholding or withdrawing food and water was equal to introducing an independent cause of death.[19] If Mr. Herbert's nutritional and hydrational needs had been met, he would have lived indefinitely, as he was not judged to be terminally ill. Mr. Herbert did not die from some underlying pathological condition, but from the lack of basic bodily resources.[20] The most disturbing features of this decision were that it destroyed the classical distinction between medical treatment and care and it denied that medical professionals had obligations to provide life-sustaining nutrition and fluids to patients in some cases when their provision would sustain human life at minimal burden to them and at no burden to the individual receiving the nutrition and fluids.

## 2
## The Claire Conroy Case

Claire Conroy was an 84-year-old resident of the Parklane Nursing Home in Bloomfield, New Jersey, and she suffered from organic brain syndrome, diabetes, and a gangrenous left leg.[21] She was admitted to the hospital in July, 1982, where her physician recommended amputation of her gangrenous leg.[22] Her nephew, Thomas Wittemore, appointed legal guardian in 1979, refused to consent to this operation, but Miss Conroy survived and was then admitted to the Parklane Home in November, 1982.[23]

After some time, her organic brain syndrome worsened, and she lost her ability to walk, speak, and/or feed herself, even though

---

[19] *Ibid.* Also see: Horan and Grant, *Legal Aspects*, P. 605.

[20] The death certificate listed diffuse encephalamalacia resulting from anoxia as the cause, but had feeding been continued, he would have continued to live indefinitely.

[21] *In the Matter of Claire C. Conroy*, 98 N.J. 321, 486 A.2d 1209 (1985) P. 1217.

[22] *Ibid.* P. 1218.

[23] *Ibid.*

she could respond to commands.[24] Miss Conroy was conscious and not comatose, but she was not able to understand her environment in an intellectual manner. Because of her difficulties in swallowing, she was eventually given food and fluids through a nasogastric tube.[25] Mr. Wittemore unsuccessfully petitioned Miss Conroy's physician to remove the feeding tube which would result in her death, but Dr. Kazemi refused to accede to this request. Mr. Wittemore then filed a complaint with the Chancery Division of the Superior Court for Essex County on January 24, 1983, to remove the feeding tube.[26] After testimony by physicians, the nursing home administrator, and an ethicist, the trial court on February 2, 1983, authorized the guardian to remove the feeding tube. This decision was stayed pending appeal, but Miss Conroy expired from other causes two weeks after the court's order.[27]

An intermediate appellate court reviewed the case, reversed the decision of the trial court, and recognized not only the right of patients to refuse treatment, but also the obligations of health care professionals to give care.[28] The court stated that nothing short of a certain diagnosis of brain death, terminal illness, or irreversible coma would justify favoring the right of privacy over the state interest in preserving life.[29] In reversing the lower court, the appellate court rejected "quality-of-life" judgments:

> Put simply, to allow a physician or family member to discontinue life-sustaining treatment to a person solely because that person's lack of intellectual capacity precludes him from enjoying a meaningful quality of life would

---

[24] *Ibid.* P. 1217.

[25] *Ibid.*

[26] *Ibid.* P. 1218.

[27] *Ibid.* P. 1217.

[28] *In the Matter of Claire C. Conroy*, 190 N.J. Super. 453, 458-60, 464 A.2d 303 305-306 (N.J.Super. A.D. 1983) Pp. 313-4.

[29] 464 A. 2d P. 310.

# MEDICAL ETHICS

> establish a dangerous precedent that logically could be extended far beyond the facts the case now before us.[*sic*] In our view, the right to terminate life-sustaining treatment based on a guardian's substituted judgment should be limited to incurable and terminally ill patients who are brain dead, irreversibly comatose or vegetative, and who would gain no medical benefit from continued treatment.[30]

And the court held that feeding tubes were not "intrusive" medical treatments, but this was sharply criticized by leading scholars:

> The nasogastric tube was no more than a simple device which was part of Conroy's routine nursing care. It was not really "medical treatment" at all. In truth, Conroy was little different from the many other ill, senile or mentally disabled persons who are bedridden and cared for in nursing homes. Consequently, the bodily invasion she suffered as a result of her treatment was small, and should not be said to outweigh the State's interest in preserving life.[31]

The court asserted that nourishment did not cure disease and was not an artificial life-sustaining device. Rather, it was a basic necessity of life which caused death when withdrawn and permitted life to continue when provided until the patient died from the underlying illness or injury.[32] The court did not hold that food and water always had to be given, but rather it identified a limited number of situations in which they could be withheld from patients. The *Conroy* appellate court was more restrictive than were other courts in permitting food and water to be withheld in that it held that they could only be withdrawn or withheld if there was a certain

---

[30] *Ibid.*

[31] 464 A.2d P. 311.

[32] Barry, R, "The Ethics of Providing Life-Sustaining Nutrition and Fluids to Incompetent Patients," *The Journal of Family and Culture*, Vol. I, No. 2, Summer, 1985. P. 23.

diagnosis of brain death, irreversible coma, or imminent death.[33]

This judgment of the intermediate appellate court was partially affirmed by the New Jersey Supreme Court. In a decision handed down on January 10, 1985, it held that Claire Conroy had to be given a feeding tube, but that nursing home residents in generally similar conditions did not have to be given food and fluids.[34] The court asserted that a guardian could order nutrition and fluids withdrawn from an incompetent patient judged to be terminally ill and in unavoidable pain under the following conditions:

1. If the patient had provided some "clear and convincing evidence" during a period of competency that nutrition and fluids were to be withdrawn or withheld;[35]

2. If there was "trustworthy" evidence that the patient would want nutrition and fluids removed or withheld and that the patient was in severe and unavoidable pain, or:[36]

3. If there was no evidence of the wishes of the patient, but the judgment of the guardian and physician was that the provision of nutrition and fluids was more burdensome than beneficial.[37]

It has been claimed that the New Jersey Supreme Court came as close as a court could to saying that euthanasia was legally permissible.[38] The first criterion places virtually no limitations on the legal right to refuse medical treatment and it would permit suicide in some instances by legally permitting patients to refuse all treatments when diagnosed as incompetent and terminally ill. This criterion would not require that even minimal care be given to terminally ill patients. And the last two standards established by the court permit all medical treatments to be removed when a

---

[33] 464 A.2d P. 310.

[34] 486 A.2d P. 1243

[35] *Ibid.* P. 1229.

[36] *Ibid.* P. 1232.

[37] *Ibid.*

[38] See: "Speakers Cite Effects of Rulings on Ethics Questions," *American Medical News*, May 3, 1985, 28, 18, P. 9. This view was offered by attorney Edward Goldman.

judgment is made by the physician that an incompetent patient is experiencing pain that markedly outweighs the physical pleasure, emotional enjoyment, or intellectual satisfaction that could still be enjoyed in life. These standards bias judgments against terminal and incompetent patients because the terminally ill often have less opportunity for intellectual satisfaction and emotional enjoyment than do others. These standards were purportedly enunciated to protect the self-determination of the patient, but the court applied them in situations where the wishes of the patient could not be known, and this fact reveals the true aim of these standards. The last two standards require physicians and guardians to make very subjective judgments about the quality of life of incompetent patients, and by allowing these sorts of judgments, the court has gone quite far in legally endorsing assisted suicide and nonvoluntary mercy killing.

## 3
## The Crista Nursing Home Case

Between October, 1984, and April, 1985, at the Crista Nursing Home in Seattle, Washington, six nurses were threatened with dismissal because they did not comply with a directive from the house medical director and administrator to remove nutrition and fluids provided by feeding tubes to two elderly women who were judged to be comatose and terminally ill.[39] The nurses objected that the women were medically stable, gave some evidence of responsiveness, and appeared to have some awareness of pain.[40] One of the patients was transferred to another nursing home where the tube was removed.[41] The other patient was transferred to another wing of the Crista Home where the feeding tube was removed.[42]

---

[39] "Two Families' Decision: Letting Loves Ones Starve," *The Seattle Times/Seattle Post-Intelligencer*, April 14, 1985, P. A6, Col. 4.

[40] *Ibid*. P. A6, Col. 3.

[41] *Ibid*. P. A6, Col. 4.

[42] *Ibid*. P. A6, col. 4.

## 4
## The "Loving Arms" Case

On July 15, 1985, the Office of Health Facility Complaints of the Minnesota Health Department issued a report concerning the death of an elderly woman at Abbott-Northwestern Hospital in Minneapolis.[43] In September, 1984, 89-year-old Ella Bathhurst, who was living alone in her own apartment, fell and broke her hip.[44] She was admitted to Abbott-Northwestern where surgery was performed on the fracture, and she was then admitted to a nursing home.[45] In her nursing home, she developed a minor case of pneumonia which was treated and she became dehydrated because of swallowing problems. She was then readmitted to Abbott-Northwestern for "gentle rehydration" and the admitting physician judged her to be in "satisfactory condition".[46]

Shortly after she was readmitted, her daughter came from New Jersey to Minneapolis and apparently ordered all medical treatments removed.[47] From that point on food, fluids, diuretics, and antibiotics were withheld, despite the fact that Mrs. Bathhurst begged for water for six days after this was done. At no point was Mrs. Bathhurst declared legally incompetent and it is not clear why her physicians caused her daughter's requests to be carried out

---

[43] Investigative Report #V85-299 filed by the Office of Health Facility Complaints, Department of Health, State of Minnesota, July 12, 1985. The investigation was conducted by Mr. Arnold Rosenthal. This was called the "Loving Arms" case because of an advertisement run by Abbott-Northwestern hospital which claimed its loving arms extended to the community to bring healing and comfort.

[44] *Ibid.* P. 1.

[45] *Ibid.* P. 1.

[46] *Ibid.* Pp. 1-2.

[47] *Ibid.* P. 5.

# MEDICAL ETHICS

instead of Mrs. Bathhurst's.[48]

Her physicians were interviewed by an investigator from the Office of Health Facility Complaints and they claimed that withholding fluids was appropriate because she had developed congestive heart failure, but they did not explain why her diuretics were withheld.[49] The hospital asserted that she received appropriate care, but it did not explain why her requests for water were denied, or why she was not given painkillers when it became clear that she was in great pain from dehydration. The physicians and staff who let Ella Bathhurst die have not been prosecuted and were merely given minor reprimands.

## 5
## The Mary Heir Case

Mrs. Mary Heir was a 94-year-old woman who had a long history of severe mental illness.[50] For fifty-five years, she was a patient in a mental hospital in Middleton, New York, after which she was transferred to Beverly Nursing Home in Beverly, Massachusetts. She required thorazine to relieve delusions and a gastrostomy because of a cervical esophageal diverticulum and a hiatal hernia.[51] The gastrostomy tube was inserted in 1975, and she

---

[48] Her physicians apparently assumed she was incompetent, but nurses noted that she was alert but very hard of hearing and this may have resulted from medications she was taking.

[49] Ibid. P. 16. One of the physicians interviewed noted that there were many treatments available for congestive heart failure, but their provision was rejected by the family and that the hospital never brought up the possibility of an NG tube or gastrostomy because it was known that the family would not have consented to them. One physician claimed that the patient was not alert or oriented, but he admitted that he had not read the nurses' notes indicating that she was alert, but hard of hearing and depressed. He himself did not know when the last time was when Mrs. Bathhurst was given anything by mouth, but he did assert that on October 24, 1984 her kidney output and input was minimal. It is not clear if this resulted from a lack of fluids, however. When it was suggested that she be given slush, he asked if it was quality of life to live on slush when one was 89 years-old.

[50] *In re*. Heir, 18 Mass. App. Ct. 200, 464 N.E.2d 959(1984).

[51] Ibid. P. 201.

dislodged it on a couple of occasions, but it was reinserted or surgically reimplanted when this happened.

During the week of April 8, 1984, it was claimed that she pulled the tube out on several occasions, and difficulties involved in reinserting it required her to be admitted to Beverly Hospital.[52] Even though she cooperated with examinations, she refused to permit the tube to be reinserted, and after examination it was determined that surgery was necessary to reinsert it.[53] To obtain consent for the surgery, a guardian *ad litem* was appointed, but prior to appointment, the petitioners revised their position and asked only that thorazine be continued and that the gastrostomy not be reinserted.[54] The guardian *ad litem* advocated surgery and was joined by an attorney appointed by the probate judge.[55]

The trial and appeals courts determined that Mrs. Heir would have rejected the feeding tube if competent and they ordered the tube removed.[56] A number of other possibilities were considered and rejected as being too risky or of limited benefit for Mrs. Heir.[57] The guardian *ad litem* went back to court a month later to seek reconsideration of the decision. After hearing testimony from a number of medical experts, the court ordered surgery and the feeding tube was successfully replaced.[58] Professor George Annas pointed out that the physicians who did not want to implant the feeding tube either treated Mrs. Heir as competent patient, which

---

[52] *Ibid*. P. 202.

[53] *Ibid*. P. 202.

[54] *Ibid*. P. 203.

[55] M. Cushing, "Key Court Cases: Where are They Now?," *Amer. J. of Nursing*, Dec., 1984, P. 1469.

[56] 118 Mass. App. Ct. 200 P. 203-5.

[57] Cushing, *supra* P. 1469.

[58] G. Annas, "Let's Starve Mary Heir To Death," *Centerscope*, (Fall 1984) P. 22.

she was not, or as a resource allocation problem.[59] He claimed that the trial and appeals courts allowed a truncated burdens/benefits analysis that really required more analysis of the facts of the case to be legitimate.[60] And he asserted that the court turned her right to refuse treatment against her when this suited the interests of others who could benefit from such a decision.[61] And Annas asserted that it was grossly unfair to label patients incompetent and then use their statements to determine treatment plans.[62]

The court considered some of the burdens of feeding Mrs. Heir but it did not consider all of its benefits, and it failed to consider certain death resulting from denial of food and water as a burden. The court did not mention that she often tried to steal food from other people's trays, that she never said that she did not want to be fed, and that the evidence indicated that she pulled out the gastrostomy tube on only one occasion.[63] Annas argued that the court pretended to be protecting the rights of a mentally ill patient, but in fact it was making a statement about the rights of these patients to have access to society's resources.[64]

## 6
## The Ordeal of Mrs. Sharon Siebert

In 1959, Mrs. Sharon Siebert was crowned queen of the Minneapolis Aquatennial Festival. Seventeen years later, she was confined to a nursing facility because of severe brain damage resulting from complications following neurosurgery in the

---

[59] *Ibid.* P. 21.

[60] *Ibid.* P. 22.

[61] *Ibid.* P. 22.

[62] *Ibid.* P. 23. Had Mary said that she wanted every treatment possible, her physicians probably would have disregarded that wish as the rantings of an insane woman.

[63] *Ibid.* P. 23.

[64] *Ibid.* P. 23.

mid-1970's.[65] Her tragic life shows how medically vulnerable persons can have untold suffering inflicted upon them by those who fail to abide by the highest standards of professional conduct.

Mrs. Siebert was later taken to Canada, for surgery following epileptic seizures.[66] While there, she suffered a series of setbacks, and in 1976, she was admitted to St. Mary's Rehabilitation Center where she developed tight leg contractures, bedsores, and other ailments, probably as a result of inferior nursing care. Shortly after being admitted there, she was noticed by Ms. Jane Hoyt, a young Harvard-educated disability rights advocate who came to believe that Mrs. Siebert suffered many of her conditions because of neglect and failure to provide adequate nursing care and treatment. A struggle between Ms. Hoyt, St. Mary's Rehabilitation Center and various state, and federal agencies continued from 1977 onward concerning proper treatment for Mrs. Siebert.[67] Various complaints were filed by Ms. Hoyt about allegedly poor care given to Mrs. Siebert, and St. Mary's once had her arrested after barring her from further visits to her.[68] This ban was lifted, however, by a decision of the Minnesota Supreme Court.[69] While Ms. Hoyt was denied visiting privileges, Mrs. Siebert was denied gifts, greeting cards, and even a Bible sent by Ms. Hoyt.[70] Also during this period, Mrs. Siebert's former husband (a physician) obtained a decrease or elimination of seizure medications because he claimed she had no seizures since her surgeries in 1977, while in fact at least five seizures had been

---

[65] J. Hoyt, "Chronology of Discrimination, "*National Women's Health Network*, (March/April 1984) P. 12.

[66] *Ibid.* P. 12.

[67] *Ibid.* P. 12.

[68] *Ibid.* P. 12.

[69] "Ruling Goes Against Parents, Doctors in Resuscitation Case," *The Minneapolis Tribune*, (February 16, 1981) P. A1.

[70] Hoyt, *supra*, note 94, P. 12.

reported in her medical records.[71]

During the time that Ms. Hoyt was denied visiting privileges, Mrs. Siebert was placed under a "Do-Not-Resuscitate" order because she allegedly had not improved in four years. But in fact she remained in stable condition.[72] In December, 1980, Ms. Hoyt obtained a restraining order to remove the DNR order.[73] The court ruled that the sincere interest of Ms. Hoyt in Mrs. Siebert's wellbeing justified her standing to sue.[74]

In an affidavit submitted to the court, Mrs. Siebert's physicians testified that she was "incapable of meaningful communication".[75] Her former husband testified that her IQ was probably between six and ten and that she had the mental capacity of a paralyzed eighteen-month-old child who could not even swallow or mumble words.[76] Another doctor claimed that she would never improve and would remain equal to a mute twelve-to-eighteen-month-old child.[77] However, Ms. Hoyt videotaped evidence demonstrating Mrs. Siebert's ability to communicate by speech with those around her play games and even engage in crafts and Sharon Siebert is now an avid Minnesota Twins fan. Ms. Hoyt tried unsuccessfully to become Mrs. Siebert's legal guardian, but was denied this despite the fact that she provided far greater care for Sharon than did any member of Mrs. Siebert's family.

Mrs. Siebert suffered a great deal of neglect because many responsible for her care regarded her as lacking the necessary human qualities to warrant continued existence. Mrs. Siebert was a perfect candidate for death by "calculated benign neglect", to use

---

[71] *Ibid.* P. 12.

[72] J. Hoyt, "No Dr. Blue/Do Not Resuscitate", *Bioethics Q.*, 3, 2, (Summer 1981) P. 128.

[73] *Ibid.* P. 132.

[74] *Ruling Goes Against Parents*, Sect. A, P. 4.

[75] Hoyt, *supra* note 94, P. 12.

[76] *Ruling Goes Against Parents*, Sect. A, P. 4.

[77] *Ibid.*

Daniel Maguire's term, because she was originally judged to be without any capacity for meaningful human relationships.[78] Her tragic story shows the need for dedicated and sincere advocates such as Jane Hoyt to intervene and protect these medically vulnerable patients.

## 7
## The Elizabeth Bouvia Case

Mrs. Elizabeth Bouvia, a 28-year-old quadriplegic and victim of cerebral palsey, petitioned a court to order Riverside Hospital in Los Angeles in 1983 to permit her to starve to death while providing her with painkillers.[79] Her petition, however, was rejected. In 1986, she petitioned a court to order High Desert Hospital to withdraw a feeding tube, by arguing that she did not wish to starve herself to death but merely to be relieved of the burdens resulting from the tube's implantation.[80] The hospital argued that Mrs. Bouvia really wished to commit suicide, and it protested its removal.[81]

A three-judge panel of a California intermediate appellate court ordered the hospital not to reinsert the tube.[82] The court also held that the hospital was required to give Mrs. Bouvia the treatments she desired, even though hospital personnel disagreed with some of her medical decisions.[83] In effect, the court compelled the staff at High Desert to materially cooperate in Mrs. Bouvia's

---

[78] Maguire, Daniel, "The Freedom to Die", in Martin Marty and Dean Peerman, *New Theology No. 2.* p. 188.

[79] *Bouvia v. Superior Court.* Slip opinion. Cal.App. Ct, #B019134, April 16, 1986. P. 5.

[80] *Ibid.* P. 22.

[81] *Ibid.*

[82] *Ibid.* P. 26.

[83] *Ibid.* P. 25.

suicide should she decide she wanted to starve herself to death.[84]

The court argued that the right to refuse medical treatments was not to be restricted, even if certain death would follow from such decisions:

> All decisions permitting cessation of medical treatment or life-support procedures to some degree hastened the arrival of death. In part, at least, this was permitted because the quality of life during the time remaining in those cases has been terribly diminished to the point of helplessness, uselessness, unenjoyability and frustration. She, as the patient, lying helplessly in bed, unable to care for herself, may consider her existence meaningless.[85]

The court also compelled health care providers to comply with her treatment-refusal decisions because of her "diminished quality of life":

> It is incongruous, if not monstrous, for medical practitioners to assert their right to preserve a life that someone else must live, or more accurately, endure for '15 to 20 years'. We cannot conceive it to be the policy of this State to inflict such an ordeal upon anyone.[86]

This decision was also noteworthy because Judge Lynn Compton held that the state and the health care professions should give whatever assistance they could to help Bouvia find a quick and painless death if she should want it. In his concurring opinion, Judge Lynn Comtpon made statements that amounted to little more than pro-euthanasia propaganda:

> Elizabeth apparently has made a conscious and informed choice that she prefers death to continued existence in her

---

[84] *Ibid.*

[85] *Ibid.* Concurring opinion, Judge Lynn Compton. P. 2

[86] *Bouvia v. Superior Court.* P. 5.

helpless and, to her, intolerable condition. I believe she has an absolute right to effectuate that decision. This state and the medical profession, instead of frustrating her desire, should be attempting to relieve her suffering by permitting and in fact assisting her to die with ease and dignity. The fact that she is forced to suffer the ordeal of self-starvation to achieve her objective is in itself inhumane.

The right to die is an integral part of our right to control our own destinies so long as the rights of others are not affected. That right should, in my opinion, include the ability to enlist the assistance from others, including the medical profession, in making death as quick and painless as possible.

That ability should not be hampered by the state's threat to impose legal sanctions on those who might be disposed to lend assistance.

The medical profession, freed from the threat of governmental or legal reprisal, would, I am sure, have no difficulty in accommodating an individual in Elizabeth's situation.[87]

In light of this statement, it is very probable that we will see a case appearing in the near future where an individual will ask for a quick and painless death by means of a lethal injection. In deciding such a case, it is almost certain that the concurring opinion of Judge Compton will be invoked to justify such measures. What this study suggests is that "aiding" terminally ill patients to die in fact exploits their despair, helplessness, and dependency.

## 8
## The Case of Mr. Paul Brophy

Mr. Paul Brophy was a 47-year-old firefighter and emergency medical technician from Easton, Massachusetts, who suffered a

---

[87] *Ibid*. P. 22.

cerebral hemorrhage and lapsed into a stupor in March, 1983.[88] It was contended in a civil case brought to the Probate court of Norfolk County that he was in a permanently vegetative state. The petition, brought by his wife, argued that the feeding tube should be removed because he was comatose with no prognosis of recovery.[89] Contrary to this view, however, medical experts examined Mr. Brophy and determined that he had a certain level of responsiveness. When a hair was waved under his nose, he turned his head violently aside, as he did when he was exposed to noxious odors.[90] He also reacted to more subtle forms of pain, and he went through sleep and wake cycles.

Judge David Kopelman rejected the petition to remove the feeding tube because Mr. Brophy was medically stable and not terminally ill. Feeding him through the tube was considered an aspect of normal, customary, and routine nursing care. Even further, Judge Kopelman noted that if feeding were to be removed, he would experience a very painful death that could be avoided by simple measures. Even further, he found that the decision to remove feeding was not intended to spare pain and suffering, but to terminate life.[91]

This case was appealed to the Supreme Judicial Court of Massachusetts which overturned the lower court decision and permitted the Brophy family to admit Mr. Brophy to a facility which would remove his feeding tube.[92] After saving a person who was badly burned in an automobile accident, Brophy purportedly said, "I don't ever want to be on a life-support system", and "when your

---

[88] Commonwealth of Massachusetts, The Trial court, The Probate and Family Court, Norfolk Division, #85E0009-G1, *Patricia E. Brophy, Guardian of Paul E. Brophy, Sr. vs. New England Sinai Hospital, Inc.* Judgment, Pp. 4-5.

[89] *Ibid.* P. 1.

[90] *Ibid.* P. 12.

[91] *Ibid.* P. 33.

[92] *Brophy v. New England Sinai Hospital,* Inc, No. 84-4152, slip op. (Mass. Sup. Jud. Ct. Sept 11, 1986) Also see: *Nota Bene,* "Brophy v. New England Sinai Hospital", in *Issues in Law and Medicine,* Vol 2, No. 3, November, 1986, p. 221. "Ruling Allows Comatose Man to Die", *The Boston Globe,* September 12, 1986. p. 1.

ticket is punched, its punched."[93] The court accepted that statement as an expression of his wishes concerning the provision of medical treatment and it ordered feeding stopped. That the court did this is remarkable because this statement expresses a suicidal wish which should not be accepted by any court. Even further, the court failed to note that Mr. Brophy regained consciousness after the aneurysm and prior to the surgery and that during that period of consciousness he never stated his wishes in any clear manner on the provision of "life-sustaining measures".[94] It was quite possible that Brophy was in the "locked-in syndrome" in which he was able to experience his environment but unable to respond to it. Justices Nolan, O'Connor and Lynch argued strongly against the decision of the majority, and one court reporter said that the Justices were more bitter toward one another than he had ever seen them in many years of court reporting.[95]

In an article in the magazine *Massachusetts Medicine* it was reported that Brophy did not die from the withdrawal of the feeding tube, because it was never taken out.[96] Instead, Easton hospital simply stopped feeding him. Thus, in the last analysis, it was not the tube that was a medical treatment, but food itself. If there is anything that shows the emptiness and fraudulent character of the "right to die" arguments it is this case, for Brophy died not because a medical treatment was withdrawn, but because he simply was not fed.

This case was crucial because it showed that proponents of mercy killing were not primarily interested in ending the suffering of the terminally ill, but in ending the lives of the medically stable who caused others to suffer. There was no sound reason to believe

---

[93] Lebowitz, Lawrence, J. "Brophy Revisited" in *Massachusetts Medicine*, Jan/Feb 1987. Pp. 11.

[94] *Letter for Petition for Rehearing Pursuant to M.R.A.P. 27*, p. 3, by Peter Gubellini. Mr. Gubellini was the attorney representing New England Sinai Hospital and he brought this fact to the attention of the Court because it had been ignored in its decision.

[95] "Ruling Allows Comatose Man to Die", *The Boston Globe*, September 12, 1986. P. 1.

[96] See: Lebowitz, Lawrence, J. "Brophy Revisited". P. 11.

that Brophy suffered from assisted feeding in his state, and the decision to remove the feeding tube seems to have been made to end his family's suffering.

## 9
## In the Matter of Beverly Requena

In April, 1985, Beverly Requena was admitted to Riverside Hospital in Denville, New Jersey, suffering from amnyotrophic lateral sclerosis.[97] While hospitalized there, she made it clear that she would not want her life to be maintained with artificial feeding.[98] Prior to that date, however, Riverside hospital merged with St. Clare's hospital, and Mrs. Requena came under the control of the Catholic hospital. St. Clare's adopted a policy in September 1986 of not removing feeding tubes from patients, and in September, 1986, she began to loose weight, and physicians wanted to insert a feeding tube to sustain her weight.[99] At that time, her family petitioned a New Jersey Court to restrain the hospital from continuing feeding.[100] St. Clare's stated that it would be quite willing to transfer Mrs. Requena to another facility that would remove the tube, but it was against their policies to permit it to be removed.[101] St. Clare's issued a policy statement shortly after the

---

[97] *In the Matter of Beverly Requena*, No. P-326-86E (N.J.Super. Ct. Morris Div. September 24, 1986). P. 1.

[98] *Ibid*. P. 1-2.

[99] *Ibid*. P. 1-2.

[100] *Ibid*. P. 5-6

[101] *Ibid*. The hospital stated this because it was its policy not to withhold basic forms of care from patients. On September 11, 1986, the board of trustees unanimously adopted the following resolution:

> BE IT RESOLVED by the Board of Trustees that it does hereby reaffirm the policy of the former St. Clare's Hospital that food and water are basic human needs and that such fundamental care cannot be withheld from patients in the medical Center and that neither the Medical Center nor its personnel will participate in the withdrawal of artificial feeding and/or fluids. P. 6.

merger, but the court argued that such a policy should not be allowed to govern Mrs. Requena's treatment.[102] The trial court held that moving her to another facility would cause her unnecessary suffering and burden, despite the fact that she was comatose at the time.[103] This decision was upheld by an appeals court hours after the case was heard in an unusual move which argued that moving her would be a psychological and emotional blow to Mrs. Requena.

On appeal, Judge David Furman held that St. Clare's policy of not withdrawing food and water from patients was valid and enforceable only if it did not interfere with the patient's right to die decision and other protected interests. Even further, he held that:

> Even if the policy embodied in the resolution is generally to be applied, application should be limited to the circumstances where it is reasonable and equitable to apply it without undue burden to the patient.[104]

Neither court actually struck down the policy of the hospital, but they held it to be inapplicable because St. Clare/Riverside Hospital did not present a suitable and convenient alternative.[105] This itself is outrageous, claiming that an institution that chooses not to participate even materially in what it considers to be a homicidal act must present a "suitable and convenient" alternative to what it believes to be morally reprehensible. It is not as if the hospital had double dealt Mrs. Requena by not informing her of its policy on feeding until she had been there for fifteen months, for she had not asked about it until she had been there for fifteen months.

---

[102] *Ibid.* P. 7-9.

[103] *Ibid.* The court agreed that Mrs. Requena could be easily moved to St. Barnabas hospital and that she would not suffer greatly from that move. It also agreed that moving her to an other facility would not cause great suffering for her family. However, it claimed that she would suffer psychologically because she would be separated from the health care providers upon whom she had become dependent and for whom she had developed a great deal of affection. For this reason, the court rejected St. Clare's offer to transfer her to another facility. Pp. 7-9.

[104] *New Jersey Star Ledger*, Tuesday, October 7, 1986. Pp. 1, 10.

[105] *Ibid.*

# MEDICAL ETHICS

This case is significant because it shows that the right to die movement will violate the constitutional freedoms of religious institutions in order to achieve its goals.

## 10
## The Mildred Rasmussen Case

Mildred Rasmussen was a 70-year-old county care nursing home and county care patient in Tucson, Arizona.[106] She supposedly declared that she would not wish to be given assisted feeding, if she ever needed it.[107] A legal guardian was appointed for her who petitioned a court to appoint him to order feeding removed. Over the objections of a court appointed guardian *ad litem* food and water were ordered to be removed on the basis of the "substituted judgment doctrine because this was judged to be in her "best interests".[108]

This case was appealed, and during the appeal, the nasogastric tube was removed.[109] After its removal, it was discovered that she could swallow, and she was fed with a large syringe. However, she died from complications of pneumonia during the appeals process.[110] The appeals court upheld the lower court that withdrawing food and water was in her best interests, but it rejected the use of "substituted judgment" when there was no evidence upon which a guardian could base such a judgment. The appeals court argued that this judgment was supported by the right

---

[106] *Rasmussen v. Fleming*, No. 2, CA-CIV 5622, slip op. P. 2 (Ariz. Ct. App. June 25, 1986).

[107] See: *Nota Bene*, "Rasmussen v. Fleming", in *Issues in Law and Medicine*, Vol. 2, No. 3, Nov. 1986, P. 211.

[108] *Ibid*. Pp. 215-6.

[109] *Ibid*. P. 211.

[110] *Ibid*. P. 211

to privacy articulated in *Roe v. Wade*.[111] The right to privacy was not lost by incompetency, according to the court.[112] Even more startlingly, the court found that in another case where there was not a shred of evidence of what the person wanted, that food and water could be withheld because this was in the patients "best interests".[113]

The appellate court in this case said that feeding and medical treatments could be ordered withdrawn by the following individuals in the following order:

> If a person is comatose and there is no reasonable possibility that he will return to a cognitive sapient state, and if it is determined by the attending physician that the person's present condition is incurable, irreversible and there is confirmation of the person's present condition by two other physicians who have been consulted in the matter, and if a vital function of the person is being sustained by extraordinary means; then extraordinary means may be discontinued upon the direction and under the supervision of the attending physician at the request any of the individuals in the following order of priority: (1) the judicially appointed guardian of the person if such a guardian has been appointed. This should not be construed to require such appointment before a treatment decision is made. (2) The person or persons designated by the patient in writing not make the treatment for him. (3) The patient's spouse. (4) An adult child of the patient, or if the patient has more than one adult child, a majority of the adult children who are reasonably available for consultation. (5) The parents of the patient. (6) The nearest living relative of the patient. (7) If none of the above are available, then at the discretion of the attending physician, the extraordinary means may be discontinued upon the direction and under the supervision of

---

[111] *Ibid.* Pp. 212-3

[112] *Ibid.* P. 213.

[113] See: O'Steen, "Climbing Up the Slippery Slope" in *Window on the Future.* P. 77.

# MEDICAL ETHICS

the attending physician.[114]

It would not be an understatement to say that these criteria have made nonvoluntary mercy killing quite easy. There is no substantive definition of what constitutes an extraordinary means, and these criteria would permit a physician to go from one individual or group to another to find someone who would authorize removal of treatment or feeding. And if he was not able to find anyone who would do this, the physician could then simply go ahead and withhold feeding and treatment himself, by arguing that such a decision was in the "best interests" of the patient and covered by the patient's right to privacy. This judgment made it far easier for physicians to gain authorization for mercy killing by omission, and it extended the protection offered by the law to mercy killers.

## 11
## The Hector Rodas Case

On January 22, 1987, Guatemalan-born illegal alien Hector Rodas was given the right by Judge Charles Buss of the Mesa County District Court in Grand Junction, Colorado to starve himself to death.[115] Mr. Rodas, who was the father of two small children, suffered total paralysis after an accident in February 1986. Physicians at the Hilltop Rehabilitation Hospital in Grand Junction, Colorado implanted a gastrostomy because of his inability to swallow, and in the summer of 1986 he petitioned the hospital to withhold feeding. The hospital did not act on his petition for a long time and then petitioned a court to determine if he was competent to make the decision. Judge Buss declared that he was competent, and he ordered feeding withheld January 23, 1986. On January 30, 1986, the Colorado ACLU filed a suit requiring the hospital and Mr. Rodas' physician to give him a lethal injection. This suit was based on statements Mr. Rodas made during the trial that he would like medications to quickly end his suffering. However, shortly after the

---

[114] *Rasmussen v. Fleming.* Pp. 16-7.

[115] "Quadriplegic now has 'Freedom' to Starve Himself", *Colorado Springs Gazette-Telegraph*, January 24, 1987. P. B8, cols. 1-6.

suit was filed, a reporter from a Grand Junction newspaper interviewed Mr. Rodas and discovered that he did not wish a lethal injection. This was reported the next day, and following that report, the ACLU withdrew it suit and requested that the court records be sealed.

The tube which Mr. Rodas protested so strongly against, however, was never removed, and like Paul Brophy, food and water were simply withheld from him.[116] It is clear from this decision that the invasive treatment that Mr. Rodas and his attorneys from the American Civil Liberties Union wanted removed was simply nutrition and hydration and not anything that required medical or even nursing skills to provide. Rodas would have lived indefinitely with the mere provision of food and water.

Mr. Rodas died on February 7, and shortly after that the Colorado ACLU filed suit against the hospital and Mr. Rodas' physician charging them with battery for having fed him prior to the trial. It is clear that the purpose of this suit was to intimidate health care givers and facilities to force them not to feed patients unless they explicitly request it. A remarkable feature of this decision was that the court did not invoke the interests of his two young children in order to prohibit him from committing suicide.[117] The intent of the actions of the ACLU suit in this case was clear: to make offering food and drink to the needy a criminal act if a person refuses it.

## 12
## The Case of Mrs. Nancy Ellen Jobes

In 1980, 25-year-old Mrs. Nancy Ellen Jobes was involved in an automobile accident while pregnant.[118] Shortly after the accident, her unborn child succumbed, and physicians attempted to remove the dead child by means of Caesarean section. Mrs. Jobes

---

[116] *Hector O. Rodas v. Hilltop Rehabilitation Hospital, et al.* Civil Action No. 87-187.

[117] It has been the usual custom of courts to place the needs and rights of minor children over the rights and needs of competent adults in such situations.

[118] *In The Matter of Nancy Ellen Jobes,* Superior Court of New Jersey, Chancery Division, Morris County. *C-4971-85E.* P. 2.

suffered a medical catastrophe and lapsed into a stupor.[119] She was admitted to Lincoln Park Nursing Home in Morristown where she was fed by a nasogastric tube, then a gastrostomy tube.[120]

In 1985, her husband and parents petitioned a court for permission to remove the feeding tube, arguing that she was in a persistent coma and would never have wanted to live the way she was living.[121] Expert witnesses summoned by the nursing home argued that she was not in a persistent coma, but was rather severely brain damaged. Dr. Maurice Victor examined her and noted that she was able to track people with her eyes and was able to lift her head from the pillow to do so.[122] He noted that she moved her head violently aside when a feather was waved under her nose or when she was exposed to noxious odors.[123] Frequently on command, she was able to wiggle her toes and he also noted a change in facial expression when she attempted to do this.[124]

On April 23, 1986, Judge Robert Stein ordered the feeding tube removed, on the ground that doing so was in accord with her expressed wishes.[125] This opinion was not in harmony with the *Conroy* standards, however, for her wishes were not stated in a living will, and she was not in severe or intractable pain. Even further, she was not an elderly nursing home patient in a terminal condition which prohibited the *Conroy* standards from applying to her, and was not expected to die within a year.[126] To justify his

---

[119] *Ibid.* P. 2.

[120] *Ibid.*

[121] *Ibid.* P. 9-11.

[122] Private communications, Dr. Maurice Victor, M.D., Department of Neurology, Case Western Reserve University to Mr. Richard Traynor, Dec. 12, 1985.

[123] *Ibid.*

[124] *Ibid.*

[125] *In the Matter of Nancy Ellen Jobes.* P. 12.

[126] *Ibid.* P. 12.

opinion, Judge Stein cited Justice Handler's somewhat question begging opinion that pain should not be taken into consideration because that would bar removal of treatments in most if not all cases.[127]

In a decision which also included the cases of Hilda Peters and Eileen Farrell, the New Jersey Supreme Court decided that the rights of terminally ill persons to reject not only medical treatments but also assisted feeding had priority not only over the interests of the state, but also over the policies of institutions.

This decision was alarming because it will have wide ranging effects on the medically vulnerable and health care institutions. The decision significantly modified the judgment of the Court in the *Claire Conroy* case and it held that a patient did not have to be in severe and untreatable pain for others to remove all care and medical treatment. Jane Hoyt, co-chair of the medical issues task force for the United Handicapped Federation, said:

> As advocates for the disabled, we are outraged by the decision, which appears to justify death on the basis of severe disability. It is active euthanasia to withdraw her successful nourishment in order to kill her by starvation.

The New Jersey Catholic Conference filed an *amicus curiae* brief in the case, and this brief is the most important statement by Catholic bishops in the U.S. on this issue to date. The bishops said that:

---

[127] Judge Stein stated:

> The court's concentration on pain as the exclusive criterion in reaching the life-or-death decision in reality transmutes the best-interests determination into an exercise of avoidance and nullification rather than confrontation and fulfillment. In most cases the pain criterion will dictate that the decision be one not to withdraw life-prolonging treatment and not to allow death or occur naturally. First, pain will not be an operative factor in a great many cases [because of the ability to reduce pain through the use of drugs]...Further,...health care providers frequently encounter difficulty in evaluating the degree of pain experienced by a patient. Finally, "[o]nly a minority of patients...have substantial problems with pain..." Thus, a great many cases, the pain test will become an absolute bar to the withdrawal of life-support therapy. *Id.* at 12-3.

> ...nutrition and hydration, being basic to human life, are aspects of normal care, which are not excessively burdensome, that should always be provided to a patient. Nutrition and hydration are directed at sustaining life. Medical treatment is therapeutic; nutrition and hydration are not, because they will not cure any disease. For that fundamental reason we insist that nutrition and hydration must always be maintained. As the Pontifical Academy of Sciences noted in this respect in its report on "The Artificial Prolongation of Life and its Exact Determination of the Moment of Death": "If the patient is in a permanent coma, irreversible as far as it is possible to predict, treatment is not required, but *care, including feeding, must be provided*.[128]

The brief also repeated a statement from the Bishops Committee for Pro-Life Activities of the National Conference of Catholic Bishops:

> Because human life has inherent value and dignity regardless of its condition, every patient should be provided with measures which can effectively preserve life without involving too grave a burden. Since food and water are necessities of life for all human beings, and can generally be provided without the risks and burdens of more aggressive means for sustaining life, the law should establish a strong presumption in favor of their use.[129]

The bishops argued that these conditions were in accord with the amendments to the federal "Child Abuse Prevention and Treatment Act", and they said that this view was endorsed by Surgeon General C. Everett Koop who said on the issue of feeding medically dependent infants that:

---

[128] Brief, *Amicus Curiae* and appendix, *In the Matter of Nancy Ellen Jobes*, on behalf of the New Jersey Catholic Conference, #26,041. P. 5.

[129] *Ibid.* P. 5

. . .the bottom line in all these cases is that you must nourish the patient (severely handicapped newborn infants). Whether an infant is in a hospital is denied food and care, or whether an infant is at home is denied food and care, the result is the same; it is child abuse.[130]

The brief quoted Professor Gilbert Meilander who said the following:

. . .deprive a person of food and water and she will die as surely as if we had administered a lethal drug, and it is hard to claim that we did not aim at her death".[131]

He also said that:

For the permanently unconscious person, feeding is neither useless nor excessively burdensome. It is ordinary human care and is not given as treatment for any life-threatening disease. Since this is true, a decision not to offer such care can enact only one intention: to take the life of the unconscious person.[132]

The bishops argued that the assertions that food and water only prolong biological life and that there is no obligation to use them is open to challenge. They held that a living human person exists until death occurs and that it cannot be truly called mere biological life.[133] It is only certain that severely brain damaged persons cannot communicate with the outside world, but it is not

[130] *P.L.* 98-57, *U.S. Code Cong., and Adm. News*, 2927

[131] Meilander, Gilbert. "On Removing Food and Water: Against the Stream", *Hastings Center Report*, Vol. 14, December, 1986.

[132] *Ibid.* P. 13.

[133] Brief, *Amicus Curiae* and appendix, New Jersey Conference of Catholic Bishops. P. 9.

# MEDICAL ETHICS

known if they can receive communication from the outside.[134] Neither can an interior life in these individuals be ruled out.

The bishops were concerned that permitting withdrawal of food and water from the comatose would put us on a slippery slope where food and water would be withdrawn from Alzheimer's patients in the near future, and they noted that some are now urging that it be withdrawn from those who are merely "pleasantly senile".[135] They also defended the right of Parklane Nursing Home not to be forced to cooperate in a decision which was contrary to their policy. And they objected to the New Jersey Supreme Court's demand that a Catholic hospital have a feeding tube removed from a woman who suffered from Lou Gehrig's disease, but this will be discussed later.

On June 24, 1987, in a 100-page brief, the New Jersey Supreme Court utterly rejected the brief submitted by the Catholic bishops and declared that the right to die is so all-encompassing that it could not conceive of a situation in which the interests of the state could override it. The Court ordered the Lincoln Park Nursing Home to remove the tube, and in an amazing display of courage before judicial arrogance, the home refused to do so. As a result, Mrs. Jobes was transferred to Morristown Memorial Hospital where she succumbed to dehydration on August 7, 1987.[136] This decision preserved some of the requirements established by the *Conroy* court, but it virtually abolished the "objective criterion" standard as being too restrictive. What this decision means is that in addition to using severe and intolerable pain as an excuse to eliminate the medically vulnerable, now strictly "quality for life" judgments made by others can be used to bring death to incompetent medically vulnerable patients. In this decision, the court has frankly condoned

---

[134] *Ibid.* P. 9.

[135] *Ibid.* Pp. 9-10.

[136] See: Hentoff, Nat. "The American Death Squads", *The Village Voice,* August 26, 1987, p. 34. Hentoff excoriates advocates of starving and dehydrating patients to death as part of the newly developing "death with dignity brigade". Hentoff argues that doctors have a duty to fight for the lives of their patients, and he cited an anti-euthanasia group as saying in all truth that "[I]t is now a capital offense to be young, brain damaged - and too tenacious to die."

nonvoluntary mercy killing because there is virtually no firm evidence that Nancy Ellen Jobes ever wanted to be brought to death by dehydration. The vague statements she purportedly made cannot suffice as evidence of her true wishes. The court has put medically vulnerable persons in grave danger from their families in this decision.

In this decision, we have the third in a year in which a court has ordered a health care institution to cooperate in the removal of nutrition and hydration from a patient when this was against its policy. The New Jersey Supreme Court is displaying remarkable arrogance in forcing individuals to act against their own consciences and in compelling institutions to violate their own policies. The decision is dangerous because it is implying that the state has no interest in preventing a wide range of patients from deliberately ending their lives when they are medically stable. The court asserted that decisions concerning the provision of medical treatments are wholly private decisions, and the interests of the state or other parties are not to dominate. "They are not to be decided by societal standards of reasonableness or normalcy. Rather, it is the patient's preferences -- formed by his or her unique experiences -- that should control". This can be construed to mean that neither family members nor the state can halt a decision by a private person that is judged to be suicidal. The decision purports to protect the right of individuals to determine the course of medical care by allowing surrogates to make decisions. But it failed to see that in the event of incompetence, whatever that might be, it is the surrogate and not the patient who is making the medical decisions. There were no clear and certain indications in Mrs. Jobes's life that she wanted to be dehydrated or starved to death, but it was clear that her family wanted her dead because they objected to the "quality of life" she experienced.

The court has granted a virtual writ of immunity to health care professionals and family members who withdraw care and treatments from patients when there is virtually no evidence of the patient's wishes. It permits surrogates "acting in good faith" however that can be determined in these cases, to order withdrawal of medical treatment and food and water from patients judged to be "terminal" or "incompetent". This decision will make it possible for AIDS patients, medically stable stroke victims and quadriplegics to end their lives on request. It will make it much easier for badly brain damaged nursing home patients to be eliminated by their families or guardians.

Some would contend that the courts are merely extending the right to privacy. I as well as others cannot take such a benign view of this situation. The mercy killing movement is seeking to make the right to end one's life's as fundamental a right as the right to abortion, a right that cannot be limited by any other interest. The court is withdrawing its protection from the medically vulnerable and abandoning them to their families. We should not believe that family's will always and everywhere treat their elderly and disabled members benignly, for it was the parents of Bloomington Baby Doe who wanted the child dehydrated to death. The disabled and incompetent of our society need the protections of law to be protected from those who have an interest in their early demise, and American courts are neglecting this obligation.

In the Rodas, Requena and now the Jobes cases, health care facilities protested withdrawal of of feeding and were ordered to do this despite their objections. We are seeing the development of a trend which aims at abolishing all individual rights in the face of the right to die. The right of the health care profession to perform its duties as it sees is being overridden by the right to die, as are rights of conscience and religious rights. The right to die is quickly being formulated by these courts as a basic and fundamental right, closely akin to the way in which the right to abortion has been formulated as a basic and fundamental right.

## 13

## The AMA Statement on Feeding the Comatose

In March of 1986, the Judicial Council of the American Medical Association announced its opinion that the withdrawal of assisted feeding from nonterminal patients who were judged to be imminently dying or terminally ill should not be considered to be unethical.[137] According to Dr. Nancy Dickey, M.D., the AMA was not promoting mercy killing, but was only talking about

---

[137] "Court Paves Way to Remove Artificial Feeding", p. 1.

"withdrawing the technology" associated with feeding.[138] One must wonder about this wooly language, for it would seem to make the refusal to throw a drowning man a life preserver withholding a life-sustaining technology. This view has received widespread approval, however, for an opinion poll sponsored by the AMA showed that 73% of those polled thought it morally unobjectionable to withdraw assisted feeding from those who were "hopelessly" ill.[139]

The mercy movement has advanced so rapidly in the United States that this position of the AMA now suggests that it has the support of the most influential profession in the nation.

## B
## THE DOCTRINES AND AIMS
## OF THE MERCY KILLING MOVEMENT

Dr. Andre Wynan, General Secretary of the World Medical Association, warned that many are promoting euthanasia to alleviate economic burdens imposed on the world health care delivery system by the world's growing elderly and infirm population.[140] A warning from such an eminent person in international medicine should not be taken lightly. That the protection of economic interests is the dominant motive for accepting the principles of situation ethics can be seen most clearly in a recent statement by Professors Arnold Arluke and Jack Levin of Northeastern University:

> The "need" to get rid of the aged has economic roots. The growing elderly population is widely regarded as a threat to the nation's budget. David B. Wilson, a Boston Globe columnist, argued that the presence of dependent elderly people is likely to "blight the experience of the young and mature". A final solution may gain support from intense job

---

[138] See: "A Deadly Serious Dilemma: Evaluating the Right to Die", in *Insight*, January 26, 1987, p. 12.

[139] See: *The Washington Times*, "73% Approve of Euthanasia", November 28, 1986, P. 5.

[140] "Euthanasia Feared as 'Solution' to Rising Health Costs", *American Medical News*, May 1, 1985, p. 3.

# MEDICAL ETHICS

competition between young and old and from demographic changes that will force fewer young workers to support the swelling numbers of elders.[141]

Dr. Jerome Marmorstein has shown that there is significant support in the medical community for the movement to deny nutrition and fluids to various classes of chronically ill patients.[142] Marmorstein, who is an editor of *Medical Tribune*, wrote that spoon-feeding elderly patients with advanced Alzheimer's disease should be considered as an extraordinary medical treatment.[143] There is a certain persuasiveness in his proposal, for spoon-feeding involves more burden for nursing personnel than does tube feeding in many instances. He also argued for "Alzheimer's Amendments" to living wills which would allow patients to order spoon-feeding withheld when a diagnosis of advanced Alzheimer's disease is made. Dr. Marmorstein seems in fact to be affirming that those who have lost their ability to control major areas of their life do not have a right to have even the simple life support of food and water.

The long range aims of some elements of the right-to-die movement were described at the recent International Conference of Right to Die Societies in Nice, France.[144] These organizations sought legalization of assisted suicide, voluntary euthanasia, nonvoluntary euthanasia, and free-standing suicide clinics.[145] The clinics were sought for those who wished to end their lives in a painless and "hygienic" manner without any accidents. They wanted to provide these for patients who were not just terminally ill, but for the "hopelessly ill", whoever they might be, and also for those who

---

[141] Arluke, A; and Levin, J. "Getting Rid of Old People", *The Minneapolis Tribune*, Sect. A, p. 19

[142] Jerome Marmorstein, M.D., "Could the New Jersey Supreme Court Decision Apply to Alzheimer's?" *Medical Tribune*, March 27, 1985, pp. 37-8.

[143] *Ibid.* P. 37.

[144] See: Rita Marker, "Pathway from Choice to Requirement", *Human Life Review*, Spring, 1985, pp. 7-8.

[145] *Ibid.* P. 8.

found life to be "meaningless".[146]

Dr. Howard Caplan expressed views about the treatment of the elderly that is clearly abusive and discriminatory against them:

> All those with advanced and chronic senility or end-stage disease should be sequestered in a separate wing (of the nursing home), with much less intervention by personnel. Treat their pain, of course. Sedate those who are noisy or combative. Allow those who refuse to eat to starve quietly instead of forcing parenteral nutrition on them. Cease all life-prolonging measures: discontinue insulin, lasix, digoxin, and all other life-sustaining medications; don't transfer any of these patients to acute-care hospitals for any reason.[147]

Attorney David Smith of Vanderbilt University argued in an address to an international ethics committee that definitions of death should be loosened so as to increase the supply of organs available for transplantation.[148] He said that "brain death" should be widened to include patients who are irreversibly unconscious, even though their brain stems are still functioning.[149] Doctors should "induce" death by withholding food and fluids, or by providing lethal injections, and Smith argued that Karen Ann Quinlan should have had death induced so that her organs could have been used more beneficially by others.[150] Clearly, Professor Smith's proposals are very close to eugenic medicine. David Mayo wrote an article summarizing recent trends in the thoughts of suicidologists and showed that there are a significant number of philosophers, ethicists and suicidologists who accept the claim that suicide can be a

---

[146] *Ibid.* P. 8.

[147] Cited in: N. Rango, "The Nursing Home Resident And Dementia" *A. of Internal Med.* (June 1985), 102. 6, P. 980.

[148] "Lawyer Calls for Looser Definition of Death to Increase Organ Supply", *National Right to Life News*, December 4, 1986, p. 4.

[149] *Ibid.*

[150] *Ibid.*

rational and moral action.[151] These views have been sharply contested, but what is significant is that a number of these reputable ethicists and suicidologists now hold that suicide can be a rational and moral action. Different arguments are presented to morally justify suicide, but most of these theorists holds that suicide is morally acceptable and rational when it prevents the prolongation of useless suffering.[152] There is much debate about what constitutes suicide as rational, but many contemporary suicidologists and ethicists hold that it is rational when suicide enables the person to minimize suffering when death is imminent. And because of this, many of them assume that these "rational" suicides are moral as well.

At its national convention in Washington in September, 1986, the Hemlock society announced the introduction of a referendum into California to legalize physician-administered lethal injections on request.[153] Apparently this course of action was taken by Hemlock because of its inability to find legislators who were willing to take the risk of being the first in our nation to introduce a voluntary mercy killing bill. The Hemlock Society sought in 1988 to amend Article 1 of the California constitution so as to include the right to "aid in dying" as a fundamental right along with the rights to life, liberty, pursuit of happiness and privacy.[154] Under the terms of this act, "terminal condition" would be defined so loosely that doctors would not have to worry about prosecution if the

---

[151] Mayo, David. "Contemporary Philosophical Literature on Suicide: A Review", in *Suicide and Ethics*, edited by Margaret P. Battin and Ronald Maris, (New York: Human Sciences Press, 1983). P. 313.

[152] *Ibid*. P. 330.

[153] Marzen, Thomas, J. "Euthanasia: On the Brink" in *Window on the Future*. P. 65.

[154] Statement by Robert Risley, co-author of the "Humane and Dignified Death Act" at *The Humane and Dignified Death Act Symposium* of the Hemlock Society on Friday, September 26, 1986. This statement was reported by Richard Doerflinger, Legislative Assistant, Pro-Life Activities Committee of the National Conference of Catholic Bishops. [Unpublished manuscript.] P. 6.

patient was not actually terminally ill.[155] This measure would allow a third party to decide on the time at which the patient would die in the event of incompetency, and the measure would protect physicians from criminal or administrative liability for giving "aid in dying".[156] Hemlock claims that there is widespread support for legalized mercy killing. It had the Roper organization conduct a poll in the spring of 1986 and the pollsters found that 62% of those polled believed that physicians ought to be legally empowered to administer "aid in dying", Hemlock's euphemism for physician-administered lethal injections on request.[157]

Dr. Pieter Admiraal spoke at the convention and said that the Dutch would probably legalize euthanasia in a broad way in the near future.[158] At the present, Dutch courts accept mercy killing if there is a firm decision, if the patient's pain is unbearable and untreatable, if mercy killing is done by the physician, and if the person is in the terminal phase of illness.[159] He said that the Dutch Royal Medical Society would publish an official book on mercy killing, and he argued that it was ridiculous to not legalize mercy killing because such legislation would prevent misuse.[160]

This move by Hemlock shows that the right to die movement does not consider itself constrained by the ordinary legislative

---

[155] *Ibid.* See Section 7187 (f). "Terminal condition" means an incurable condition which, regardless of application of life-sustaining procedures, would, within reasonable medical judgment produce death *within six months*, and where the application of life-sustaining procedures only serves to postpone the moment of death of the patient.

[156] *Ibid.* This refers to Section 7189 (b) of the Act. "There shall be no criminal, civil or administrative liability on the part of any person for failure to act upon a revocation made pursuant to this section unless that person has actual knowledge of the revocation."

[157] *The Hemlock Quarterly*, No. 24, July 1986. P. 1.

[158] Doerflinger, *art. cit.* Pp. 24-5. And in a debate with him on the ABC *Nightline* program on February 3, 1987, he contended that he would not give euthanasia to a person simply because they were in pain because pain could be treated. Rather he would give euthanasia because a person had lost his or her "dignity".

[159] *Ibid.* P. 25.

[160] *Ibid.* P. 25.

processes, but is free to pursue other avenues to achieve its goals. It recognizes that its objectives could never be attained because of the restraints placed on our legislative system. Therefore, it is attempting to legalize mercy killing by circumventing our legislative system and going directly to the people.

A study by Susan Waller of trends in public acceptance of euthanasia, showed that there was growing worldwide support for both active and passive voluntary mercy killing.[161] There is, however, uneven support for voluntary active euthanasia among young people. This is a new finding, because they have usually been less willing to support active voluntary euthanasia than have the elderly.[162] She found that in the Netherlands, two thirds of the population of that nation support voluntary mercy killing of the terminally ill, and seventy percent of the population supported legalization of mercy killing.[163]

## Conclusion

Between 1986 and 1988 the debate on the ethics of rational suicide and euthanasia fully emerged, and it is not likely that this debate will have an outcome that will further protection of the medically vulnerable. Many leading ethicists do not accept the notion that direct and intentional killing in any form is unethical, and with that view being challenged, it is hard to see how legalization of mercy killing can be stopped.[164] We re now seeing cases where nurses and doctors who respect life will be either legally forced to give lethal injections to patients or will be sued for battery for attempting to feed patients who wish to end their lives by starvation.

---

[161] Waller, Susan. "Trends in Public Acceptance of Euthanasia Worldwide", in *The Euthanasia Review*. Vol. 1, No. 1, Spring, 1986. P. 33.

[162] *Ibid*. P. 45.

[163] *Ibid*. P. 41.

[164] Mayo, "Contemporary Literature on Suicide: A Review". Pp. 327-343.

# CHAPTER FIVE
# ADVANCE DIRECTIVES AND "AID-IN-DYING": PROBLEMS AND PARADOXES

## A
## ADVANCE DIRECTIVES

Within the past five years thirty eight states have enacted various kinds of "living will" laws which purportedly permit patients to determine in advance what kinds and levels of medical treatment are to be given them in the event that they should become incompetent and terminally ill.[1] On August 8, 1986, the National Conference of Commissioners on Uniform State Laws voted 37 to 10 to approve the "Uniform Rights of the Terminally Ill Act" (hereinafter referred to as the Act).[2] The final draft of the Act was distributed by the National Conference in January, 1986, together with a Prefatory Note and Official Comments. The purpose of this chapter is to critique the terms of the Act because it stands as a model for many living wills and many points made about the Act will validly apply to other forms of advance directives.

The larger purpose of "living will" legislation--to assure that a patient's desire that treatment be foregone is honored by health-care providers after the patient is no longer able directly to make treatment decisions--was judged by the Conference to be served by this Act, and the Act went to great lengths to encourage the use of "living wills".[3]

The specific goals of the Act were stated in the Prefatory Note:

---

[1] In general, see the publications of the Society for the Right to Die for information concerning the living will. In particular, see their Handbook of Living Will Laws 1981-4, (New York: Society for the Right to Die, 1984) and their newsletters. In addition, see their *Handbook of Enacted Laws*.

[2] See: Society for the Right to Die, *Handbook of Living Wills 1981-1984*.

[3] Uniform Rights of the Terminally Ill Act 1 (Prefatory Note) (approved at annual meeting of the National Conference of Commissioners on Uniform State Laws held August 2-9, 1985). (Available from National Conference of Commissioners on Uniform State Laws at 645 N. Michigan Ave., Suite 510, Chicago, IL 60611)

The purposes of the Act are (1) to present an Act which is simple, effective, and acceptable to persons desiring to execute a declaration and to physicians and health-care facilities whose conduct will be affected, (2) to provide for the effectiveness of a declaration in states other than the state in which it is executed through uniformity of scope and procedure, and (3) to avoid the inconsistency in approach which has characterized the early statutes.

The Act's basic structure and substance are similar to that found in most of the existing legislation. The Act has drawn upon existing legislation in order to avoid further complexity and to permit its effective operation in light of prior enactments. Departures from existing statutes have been made, however, in order to simplify procedures, improve drafting, and clarify language.[4]

This Act provides a competent person of eighteen or more years of age with the power to execute at any time a declaration governing the withdrawal of life-sustaining medical treatments. Under its provisions, the declaration would go into effect if, and only if:

1. The patient executed the declaration as an adult.
2. The patient was of "sound mind" when the declaration was executed.
3. The declaration was concerned with the withholding or withdrawal of treatment.
4. The declaration was signed by the patient or another individual of the patient's direction.
5. The signature of the patient was witnessed by two "individuals".
6. The declaration was "communicated to" the patient's attending physician.
7. The patient's attending physician determined that the

---

[4] See: T. Marzen, The "Uniform Rights of the Terminally Ill Act":A Critical Analysis, *Issues in Law and Medicine*, 1, 6. 1986, 451-452.[hereinafter cited as *Analysis*]

patient had a "terminal condition".

8. The patient's attending physician determined that the patient was "no longer able to make decisions" concerning life-sustaining treatment.[5]

The Act does not explicitly contain any provisions that would protect the right of the patient to *receive* treatments.[6] It considers food and fluids to be a medical treatment, and it permits patients to order their withdrawal when a diagnosis of terminal illness and incompetency is established.[7] It does not require that reasonable standards be employed to establish diagnoses of terminal condition or incompetency and it does not require that the patient be informed of such a diagnosis.[8] The requirement of the Act that only a competent adult be permitted to execute a declaration refusing treatment in certain cases is little more than a symbolic gesture because there is no requirement imposed by the Act to verify the majority or mental competence of the declarant at the time of execution. The Act does not impose any requirements on witnesses, and it would be technically possible for a psychotic child to be a witness to the signing of a living will.

The Act is outrightly lax in the requirements it imposes on physicians. The only standard to be applied to determine if a patient is truly terminally ill is the subjective standard of the judgment of the physician.[9] The Act relieves physicians of the usual duty to provide treatments to incompetent patients, not because of difficulties involved in obtaining informed consent, but because of a "shot in the dark" prior refusal to accept any medical treatments.[10] It does not require that the declarant be informed of treatment

---

[5] *Ibid.* P. 444.

[6] *Ibid.* Pp. 468-70.

[7] See: R. Marker, Controversial Uniform "Living Will" Act Approved, *Human Life Issues*, 1 (Supp, Fall 1985).

[8] Marzen, *Analysis*, Pp. 472-3.

[9] *Ibid.* P. 445.

[10] *Ibid.* P. 445.

alternatives as would generally be done in order to permit informed consent, and the physician does not have to be involved for a declaration to be valid.[11] And because of its ambiguity, the physician would be provided with an authority broad enough to render a declaration inoperative at will.[12]

The Act only addresses the issue of withdrawing or withholding treatment from incompetent terminally persons, and in so doing, it addresses the least controversial issues of treatment of the ill and incompetent.[13] The knotty problem of exactly how much treatment to provide a competent terminally patient is completely ignored by the Act, as is the question of how minors or persons with nonterminal conditions are to be treated.[14] And a decision to forego treatment in other difficult situations, such as permanent coma or vegetative states, is also neglected.[15]

Despite its failure to broach these questions, the Act does take some controversial stands. For example, the it prohibits taking insulin from an incompetent person who has signed a declaration because it does not consider diabetes a terminal condition.[16] Yet it permits food and water to be withdrawn from patients who will die "in a relatively short period of time". It thus regards food and water as a medical treatment that treats some types of terminal conditions.[17] But if that is the case, then why then should not

[11] *Ibid*. P. 445

[12] *Ibid*.

[13] *Ibid*. Pp. 445-6.

[14] *Ibid*.

[15] *Ibid*. P. 462.

[16] *Ibid*. P. 464.

[17] *Ibid*. P. 461. Marzen states: "The plain language of the definition of "terminal condition" states that a "condition" may be *either* incurable *or* irreversible in order to qualify as "terminal" (so long as the condition would result in death without the use of "life-sustaining treatment"). This disjunctive construction in the language of the Act is flatly contradicted by the Comment, which states that "the phrase 'incurable *or* irreversible' is to be read as circumstances warrant". P. 461. Marzen then rightly asks

spoon-feeding also be considered as a medical treatment that could be withdrawn or withheld in some instances as well?

One would think that the narrowness of the scope of the Act would give it a great deal of precision, but this is not the case. It allows medical treatments to be removed from "terminally ill patients", even if their terminal condition is reversible.[18] By allowing terminally ill patients to forego life-sustaining medical treatments, a patient could easily understand this to mean a respirator in the case of cancer. But it could also include either antibiotics for infection or nasogastric feeding, and one must wonder if patients who sign withdrawal of treatment declarations really are intending to do this.

By executing a declaration under the terms of the Act, the patient faces irresolvable ambiguities.[19] The Act aims at protecting the decision-making authority of competent patients after they have lost competence, but the lack of safeguards places that authority into serious jeopardy. It seems that the safeguards ordinarily included in other "living will" acts were excluded in order to facilitate the execution of uniform living wills.[20] The Act does not impose any material or objective standards for determining that a patient is terminally ill, and thus a physician could forego making such a judgment and could continue to treat the patient aggressively right up to the moment of death.[21]

Further, when a physician learns of the existence of a living will after he makes a determination that the patient is terminal, the only option he would have to executing the declaration would be to

what the conditions would be that would warrant such a conjunctive construction.

[18] Marzen discusses these ambiguities quite well in his article at 451-470 where he shows the tautologies involved in the Act's understanding of the critical terms "terminal condition", "relatively short period of time" and "life sustaining treatment".

[19] The only safeguards that remain are *ex post facto* criminal penalties that do not protect against the possibility that the patient was incompetent or a minor at the time of execution. *Ibid*. Pp. 457-8.

[20] *Ibid*. P. 471. If a physician's judgment is made in good faith, the Act would hold that it should not then be questioned.

[21] *Ibid*. P. 453.

transfer the patient to another facility, which could operate to inhibit the practice of sound medicine.[22] This, coupled with the strict obligation incumbent upon the physician with knowledge of a living will to either transfer the patient to a physician who will remove treatments or execute the declaration, increases the prospect that an invalidly executed will would be acted upon.[23]

The Act does not explicitly allow a physician who is aware of a declaration to disregard the declaration and treat the patient according to his or her own best medical judgment. But if a physician wished to continue treating the patient, he or she could merely ignore a living will and argue that it was not clear that the patient was terminal or competent when the document was signed.[24]

The lack of safeguards for the determination of incompetency is distressing because most treatment deferral declarations are signed after a person has been diagnosed as terminally ill and these individuals are often in significant psychological and emotional distress.[25] There is no safeguard to assure that the patient truly cannot make decisions, and it is conceivable that a competent patient's decisions could be overruled by a physician who arbitrarily judged the patient to be incompetent.

Many crucial terms in the Act are defined in a very ambiguous and nebulous fashion. For example, it holds that treatments could be withheld if a patient was expected to die within a "relatively short period of time" and if their provision would "only prolong the dying process".[26] But one must ask to what events this period of time is relative?[27] And the term "relatively short period of time" is alien to law and medicine and even ethics because it is vague, ambiguous, situational, and of little guidance to the patient,

---

[22] *Ibid.* P. 456.

[23] *Ibid.* P. 472-3.

[24] *Ibid.* P. 454.

[25] *Ibid.* P. 464.

[26] *Ibid.* P. 466.

[27] *Ibid.* P. 468.

physician, or court which would have to construe its meaning.[28] But the Act holds that treatments must be provided if the patient would live indefinitely with their provision.[29] Treatments could be removed, not if death was "imminent" but only if death would come in a "relatively short period of time".[30] This could mean that patients who lapsed into a permanent coma would have to be given all medical treatments until death would come "in a relatively short period of time", and it is unlikely that a patient would execute a declaration for such a purpose.[31]

While most treatment deferral declarations described a terminal condition as one where death would be imminent whether or not life-sustaining procedures were applied, the Act chooses to hold that a terminal condition exists when a person would die "without the administration of life-sustaining treatment".[32] The result of this is that the conditions under which treatments can be removed are increased significantly. There is no absolute

---

[28] *Ibid.* P. 465. Marzen points out that the Act might very well allow treatments to be withdrawn or withheld from a patient who could live indefinitely with them, even though this is contradicted by the Comment on the Act issued by the Conference. There remains, however, evidence that treatments, such as nasogastric feeding for a persistently vegetative patient, could be withdrawn precisely because it would enable the patient to live indefinitely. *Ibid.* P. 463.

[29] On this point, Marzen states:

> The National Commissioners plainly employed this formulation in preference to others--in particular, to a requirement that death be 'imminent'--because it was believed both to encompass a greater period of time and to provide physicians with greater discretionary latitude. *Ibid.* at 466.

[30] Marzen believes that this confused state of affairs was unintentional, but one must wonder if the Commissioners were not promoting this kind of act so that it might be rejected, thereby opening the door for a Uniform Medical Power of Attorney Act that would give terminally ill patients even more authority to refuse care and medical treatments. See: *Ibid.* P. 465.

[31] *Ibid.* P. 449. In adopting this position, the Act was in harmony with the position adopted by the President's Commission for the Study of Ethical Problems in Medicine and Biomedical and Behavioral Research, *Deciding to Forego Life-Sustaining Treatment*, at 126-36.

[32] *Ibid.* P. 463.

requirement in the Act that a "terminal condition" be irreversible.[33] The "Comment" on the Act issued by the Conference also made it clear that it would be permissible to withdraw or withhold forms of treatment even if their provision would prolong life indefinitely.[34]

The Act asserts that fraud and abuse would be limited by criminal penalties for falsification or forgery of documents.[35] But it is not clear that the penalties imposed by the Act would guarantee that the patient was of sound mind at the time of execution, and obtaining evidence of coercion or fraudulent procuring of declarations would be hard to come by, particularly after the patient has died.[36] There are virtually no penalties attached to premature withdrawal of treatments, and because the patient would be dead, it would be very difficult to determine with any certainty if treatments were prematurely withdrawn.[37] The Act holds that physicians could execute a living will when the existence of the will is communicated (as by a telephone call), but it does not require that the physician investigate the competence of the patient at the time it was executed or examine the mental status of the witnesses.[38] Because of this, one wonders how much protection

[33] *Ibid.*

[34] *Ibid.* P. 450.

[35] *Ibid.* P. 455. Marzen rightly points out that it would be best to guard against these sorts of actions before treatments are withdrawn than to punish them after the act the resulting death would be an irreparable injury.

[36] *Ibid.* P. 458.

[37] *Ibid.* P. 457. Marzen believes that the lack of safeguards described here open treatment deferral declarations open to significant abuse and destroy the myth that living wills assure the decision-making authority of once competent persons. *Ibid.* P. 458.

[38] Statement on the Uniform Rights of the Terminally Ill Act, Committee for Pro-Life Activities, National Conference of Catholic Bishops, June 1986. (This may be obtained from the Office of Pro-Life Activities, National Conference of Catholic Bishops, 1312 Massachusetts Ave., N.W., Washington, D.C. 20005.) Pp. 5-6. The National Conference of Catholic Bishops has not outrightly condemned "living wills", but they have expressed a number of grave reservations about them because of the way in which they are being promoted by euthanasia advocacy organizations. Their refusal to condemn living wills is mystifying to some Catholics particularly in light of the fact that the National Conference

against fraud and abuse the Act really affords.

In a statement issued in June, 1986, the National Conference of Catholic Bishops was critical of the Uniform Rights of the Terminally Ill Act, and they also found that the Act raised new and troubling moral problems.[39] The bishops upheld the teaching that one had to use "ordinary" means to preserve life--means which could effectively preserve life without imposing grave burdens on the patient--and they asserted that the failure to apply those means was equivalent to euthanasia.[40] However, the bishops defended the right of patients to refuse "extraordinary" medical treatments which involved too grave a burden for the patient.[41]

The bishops objected to the Act's overly broad extension of the right to refuse care and treatment.[42] They also protested ambiguities of the Act which would permit many medically stable patients who could live a long time with treatments to refuse these. Ambiguities that would permit patients who suffered only from disabling conditions to refuse life-sustaining treatments also prompted objections from the bishops.[43]

---

of Commissioners has positively promoted them in the "Uniform Rights of the Terminally Ill Act". Some Catholics recall that nearly twenty years ago the Conference endorsed a Uniform Abortion Rights Act that significantly promoted the cause of liberalized abortion, and they fear that the National Conference is leading the nation into euthanasia in the way that it was led into abortion by the National Conference nearly two decades ago.

[39] *Ibid*. P. 2.

[40] *Ibid*.

[41] *Ibid*. P. 9.

[42] *Ibid*. P. 5.

[43] *Ibid*. P. 6. It is regrettable that the bishops did not define the provision of life-sustaining, successful medically providable nutrition and fluids by the routine nursing procedures as an aspect of routine, customary normal nursing care. Had they done this, they would not have only been in greater harmony with the prevailing view of contemporary medical professionals but also in agreement with a report issued recently by a working committee of the Pontifical Academy for Sciences. In this report, the Academy stated that "If the patient is in permanent coma, irreversible as far as it is possible to predict, treatment is not required, but care, including feeding, must be provided." See: "Basic Care Required for Irreversibly Comatose", *Our Sunday Visitor*, Nov.

The Act was also criticized for its views on the provision of food and water, and they flatly stated that for most patients the provision of nourishment is morally obligatory even in situations when other medical treatments can be withdrawn.[44] They pointed out that food and water are necessities of life and can be provided without the grave risks and burdens that are involved in the provision of some other more aggressive forms of treatment.[45] The bishops believed that the Act permitted food and water to be removed from patients for whom they would be a great benefit, and they were also critical of the Act because it did not recognize the distinct and fundamental benefit of the provision of food and water--that of sustaining life.[46]

The bishops criticized implied or stated negative judgments in the Act about unconscious or otherwise disabled patients and denounced proposals to withhold nourishment precisely to end their lives.[47] They urged society to make greater efforts to protect the handicapped and disabled from medical abuse and neglect.[48] And they rejected the provision of the Act which would allow a woman to refuse medical treatments that would save the lives unborn children whenever she herself fulfilled the conditions set forth in the Act.[49]

The bishops objected to the Act not stating what were the legitimate state interests in preserving life, preventing suicide or homicide, protecting innocent third parties, and protecting the ethics

---

17, 1985, at 17. There are many Catholic ethicists who reject the notion that assisted feeding is an aspect of routine and customary care, and they thereby are abetting those who promote the direct killing of the comatose by starvation or dehydration.

[44] *Ibid.* P. 6.

[45] *Ibid.* P. 6.

[46] *Ibid.* P. 7.

[47] *Ibid.* P. 7.

[48] *Ibid.* Pp. 7-8.

[49] *Ibid.* P. 8.

of the medical profession.[50] They objected to broad immunities given to those who withdrew or withheld life-sustaining medical treatments.[51] In their judgment, the Act was also defective because it did not encourage communication between the patient and physician.[52] It tended to exclude family members from the decision-making process, and the vagueness of the Act's language gave the patient little indication of the broad power to remove life-sustaining medical treatments allotted to others in living wills.[53]

The Uniform Rights of the Terminally Ill Act claims that it permits patients to control medical decisions when they are incompetent. However, when the patient is incompetent, it is not the patient who is making the medical decisions, but the physician, guardian or family member. However, it is the physician who determines if the patient is competent or incompetent merely sick or actually terminally ill actually has full control of the medical decisions of the patient. It is the physician who has full control over the medical treatment of the patient because the physician determines if the treatments are ordinary or extraordinary and thus to be provided. When the final decisions are made, the patient has nothing to say about when the treatments are withdrawn or provided.

The Act imposes no demand that the patient be informed either before the living will is being executed, or after it has been executed. If it were to be executed, it would then be presumed that the patient was incompetent, and demands of the patient that the will be invalidated could be dismissed. More interestingly, the Act violates the ethical requirements of informed consent. These requirements demand that the patient be informed of the precise and specific treatment it is that they are being asked to give their consent to and there is no way in which a person who signs a living will can know to what the exact treatments are to which they are

---

[50] *Ibid.* P. 9.

[51] *Ibid.* P. 9.

[52] *Ibid.* P. 9.

[53] "Euthanasia Feared as "Solution" to Rising Health Costs," *American Medical News*, (May 17, 1985) P. 3.

giving consent. The Uniform Rights of the Terminally Ill Act does not specify the treatments that are being rejected when one is incompetent and terminally ill, and this violates informed consent. It misrepresents living wills to say that the patient controls the medical decisions because the health care provider makes these decisions. It is not the patient who decides any of these questions.

The Act purports to be protecting the patient from overtreatment or undertreatment, but it is the physician who is in fact most fully protected in any medical decision he or she makes. If a physician decides not to remove a medical treatment, it can simply be claimed that a diagnosis of terminal illness is not justified. But if a decision is made to remove treatments, it can be rationalized after the fact by asserting that the patient was terminally ill. Under the stipulations of the Act, there is no requirement that there be clear and convincing evidence of a living will. All that is required for a physician to execute a living will is that a phone call be placed in which someone verifies the existence of the living will.

The Uniform Rights of the Terminally Ill Act permits suicide in some cases, and in that respect it violates the duty of the state to protect the medically vulnerable from themselves. A person who needed minor medications could forego them, and there would be nothing that the state could do to prevent such a person from committing suicide. The Uniform Rights of the Terminally Ill Act would also violate the ethical duties and obligations of health care professionals because their duty is to care and cure. But living wills that are based on the pure contentless autonomy model of patient decision making could force health care providers to materially cooperate in actions that violate their professional ethical duties. For example, in situations where readily available and nonburdensome medical treatments could readily sustain life, such as in the case of Hector Rodas, health care professionals could be forced to cooperate in acts by a court that the professionals believed violated their codes of ethics, and this would violate their consciences and the ethical principles of the profession.[54] This could seriously undermine health care professionals as it would punish

---

[54] See: Jay, M.D., Allen. "The Judge Ordered Me to Kill My Patient", *Medical Economics*, August 10, 1987. Pp. 120-124.

aggressive treatment of illness, and compensate and protect lackadaisical attitudes toward medical practice.

It is hoped that these remarks will demonstrate some of the serious difficulties involved with living wills and advance directives. It is by no means clear that living wills could prevent overtreatment or undertreatment, but the *Hemlock* Society believes that they would be appropriate for authorizing voluntary mercy killing, and it first proposed that euthanasia by legalized by simply appending euthanasia language to the California Natural Death Act.[55] In Holland, the majority of patients who received euthanasia in 1985 requested it by means of a living will. Living wills can readily promote mercy killing, but it is not clear that they can do anything else effectively.

## B
## AID IN DYING

At its national convention in 1986, the *Hemlock* Society announced that it would introduce a referendum into California that would legalize physician-administered lethal injections upon request to terminally ill patients. On September 23. 1987, the California Bar Association passed a resolution supporting this sort of legislation by a margin of 282 to 239.[56]

The widespread support indicated in the Roper Organization poll of Californians, showing that 62% of Protestants and 58% of Catholics polled supported giving physicians the legal power to end the life of a terminally ill patient shows that mercy killing is becoming quite popular.[57] It also shows that many people have not thought critically about the consequences of legalizing physician-administered lethal injections on request. In this section, I wish to point out some of the practical problems and paradoxes

---

[55] See: "Doctors Cool to California Proposal to Allow 'Physician-Assisted Death'". *Physicians Financial News*, July 15, 1987. Pp. 3, 12.

[56] "Lawyers' Group Backs Doctors' Aid in Suicide" *New York Times*, September 23, 1987, P. 18, col. 1.

[57] See: Humphry, Derek. Ed. *Compassionate Crimes, Broken Taboos*. (Los Angeles: Hemlock Society, 1986). Pp. 85-6.

that are inherent to legalized physician-administered lethal injections. Thus, the problems and paradoxes with the *Hemlock* proposal will be discussed and analyzed.

## 1
## Euthanasia: The Educational Problem

The most serious problem with the *Hemlock* referendum is the message it would communicate to the emotionally unstable and the immature. On the ABC television program *Nightline*, Dr. Pieter Admiraal, M.D. indicated that the ideal way to give "aid in dying" was to gather the family of the person to be killed about the individual as they are to receive it.[58] This would show to the individual receiving "aid in dying" that they were not being abandoned, but that the action was being done out of love, compassion and support.

This scenario points out the serious educational problem that legalized euthanasia would present. In either very blunt and crude ways or in much more subtle ways, legalized and socially endorsed "aid-in-dying" would communicate a message to the immature and emotionally unstable that the rational and intelligent way of coping with grave suffering or loss of dignity would be to deliberately end one's life. Dr. Admiraal wishes to limit "aid-in-dying" to those who are rational, emotionally stable, competent and in control of their lives.[59] But limiting self-killing to them alone would communicate to the immature and emotionally unstable that suicide was the way for those who are emotionally mature to cope with suffering, a message we do not wish to communicate to our young today.

We should also recall that the immature and the emotionally unstable do not perceive reality in the same way that the mature, rational and competent do. The immature and unstable are often not able to see the fine distinctions and subtle reasons that the mature, competent and rational see. They tend to act impulsively and without due consideration in many circumstances, and when they perceive their elders electing to end their lives when they

---

[58] February, 3, 1987.

[59] *Ibid.*

experience suffering, they will see this as a warrant to end their own lives but on their own terms.

At this time in America, we need to communicate that they are not to deliberately harm themselves to cope with suffering. We wish to teach them that they are not to take drugs, smoke, engage in frivolous sexual encounters, or kill themselves to resolve the problems of alienation, loneliness, suffering and anxiety. But if they see their elders who are supposedly wise, mature and intelligent killing themselves to escape their sufferings, it will be difficult if not impossible to persuade them not to imitate them.

## 2
## Overturning the Common Law Tradition

Another serious problem with legalizing "aid-in-dying" is that it would overturn the common law tradition on homicide. This tradition has consistently prohibited acts such as giving "aid-in-dying" because these acts are deliberate and willful killings of innocent sick, despairing, disabled, and dying private citizens by other private citizens. The common law tradition has also objected to legalized voluntary mercy killing because the motive of a homicidal act not done in self-defense has never been permitted as an excuse for the act. The common law tradition has seen that if altruistic motives were allowed to excuse homicidal acts, then one would be logically committed to permitting such motives for killing the innocent as protecting the welfare of the community to justify other forms of killing of innocent private citizens.

The common law tradition has also refused to allow motives to justify killing because it is not possible in a great number of instances to determine what the motives of an individual actually are.[60] The experience of German physicians between 1920 and 1945 should remind us of how difficult this is. For, many of them during the Weimar and National Socialist eras killed energetically believing that they were acting out of laudable motives. They thought their

---

[60] This was seen most clearly in the famous case of Roswell Gilbert who was convicted of first-degree murder for the killing of his wife Emily. The jury rejected his claims that he was acting out of compassion, and convicted him because if his action, ignoring his motives. See: "Man Convicted of Killing Wife Who Begged to Die", *The New York Times*, May 10, 1985. P. 1A.

actions were wholly upright, and when the law permitted them to follow their own judgments frightful consequences followed. Medicine needs clear guidelines to direct itself to keep from being the most dangerous of all professions.[61]

Any killing that has been permitted by this tradition, with the exception of killing in self-defense, has been governed and controlled by the state so that it could bring the rigorous scrutiny of the judicial system to prevent unjust killings. Legalization of "aid-in-dying" would deny the state its classical role of protecting innocent private citizens from other private citizens, and this would be an unprecedented change in the common law tradition.

The common law tradition has adamantly opposed permitting private citizens to kill other private citizens because such actions cannot be rectified if a wrong is done. Unlike other actions such as extortion or embezzlement where there is the possibility of the damage being rectified, if an unjust act of killing occurs, there is no possible way of rectifying the damage. Legalized mercy killing would have to be subjected to the same rigorous standards that regulate capital punishment to minimize the danger of unwarranted and unjustified acts of mercy killing. Should legalized mercy killing be permitted, it would be a revolution in our common law tradition of the most profound nature.

Probably the most important reason "aid-in-dying" has been rejected by the common law tradition has been that the practice of mercy killing is fundamentally uncontrollable. This is seen by the fact that those societies which have permitted voluntary mercy killing have found that they could not keep it under effective control. ABC television reported on February 3, 1987 that nurses in Holland were being convicted of homicide for having given euthanasia to patients with out the authorization of a physician,

---

[61] This recalls the famous statement of Dr. Christoph Huhfeld:

> If the physician presumes to take into consideration in his work whether a life has value or not, the consequences are boundless and the physician becomes the most dangerous man in the state.

See: Werthem, M. D., F. *The German Euthanasia Program*, (Cincinnati: Hayes, 1973) P. 25.

which was contrary to contemporary Dutch law.[62] The euthanasia programs of Germany under the Weimar Republic and National Socialists were notorious for its lack any effective control. And in our own country, in December, 1986 Dr. Joseph Hussman was convicted in December, 1986 of mercy killing because he put a dose of Demerol in his mother's feeding tube. There was never any pretension of the act being voluntary suicide as his mother never requested this, and he killed her simply to accede to the wishes of his family. Dr. Hussman, however, was not sentenced to jail because the judge claimed that no good purpose would be served by such a sentence.[63] These all show that nonvoluntary mercy simply cannot be controlled without expanding it to such an extent that it poses grave dangers to the sick, handicapped, disabled, dying and despairing.

Advocates of "aid-in-dying" claim that they seek to limit it to the rational and those who are emotionally stable. But there is no agreement among its advocates as to what constitutes rationality. Nor is there agreement as to what classes of patients or persons should be given or denied mercy killing. For example, some wish to administer "aid-in-dying" only to those who are experience severe physical pain, while others would give it to those who believe their lives are hopeless, whatever that might mean. If either of these classes of persons are permitted to kill themselves, the other will press their claims even more vigorously. Approving it for some classes of patients will only increase pressure for it to be given to other classes of patients.

Even allowing only those who are in incurable and untreatable suffering to kill themselves eventually becomes uncontrollable. This is so because there is nothing in the principle that those who are suffering can end their lives that could restrict this to one class of patients. If self-killing were not to be allowed to a class of patients it would not be because some principle prohibited it, but merely because an arbitrary decision was made to

---

[62] ABC Television, *World News Tonight*, February 3, 1987.

[63] See: "Doctor is Spared Jail Term in Mercy Killing," *The New York Times*. December 20, 1986, p. A29-30. Even though Roswell Gilbert was convicted for killing his wife. It seems that euthanasia will be reserved to physicians in this country just as it was in Nazi Germany.

exclude them. There is no way of determining whose suffering or loss of dignity is worse than others. Is the suffering of a terminally ill cancer patient worse than that of a lovelorn adolescent? How can the law determine which of these two should have the right to commit suicide?

### 3
### "Aid-in Dying": Health Care Providers Turned Killers

Legalizing "aid-in-dying" would necessarily make killers out of healers which would undermine and compromise the objectives of the healing professions.[64] Legalized euthanasia would necessarily involve health care providers in killing because it would be necessary to use their expertise and judgment to assure that mercy killing was restricted only to those categories of patients for whom it was intended. And to use physicians for these purposes would make them formal cooperators in the killing of the sick, terminal, dying, depressed and despairing.

Legalizing "aid-in-dying" which turns healers into killers is objectionable because in the words of an Auschwitz survivor quoted by Dr. Robert J. Lifton, M.D. in his recent book *The Nazi Doctors*: "The doctor...if not living in a moral situation...where limits are very clear...is very dangerous."[65] Dr. Lifton attempted to understand from a psychiatric viewpoint how it happened that many German doctors were turned from their traditional professional goals of healing into killers for the Nazis. Lifton suggested that they engaged in a psychological process called "doubling" in which the physician created an alternate "self" who was responsible for the

---

[64] Dr. Francis Healy, M.D., a member of the California Medical Association's statewide ethics committee, made this point rather bluntly when he said about the legalization of physician-administered lethal injections: "As a physician, I take the longstanding position that you don't kill people. In the C. M. A. we've tried to preserve some consistency in doctors' roles. A doctor can't walk in one door as a healer and out another as a killer." See: "Doctors Cool to California Proposal to Allow 'Physician-Assisted Death", p. 12

[65] Lifton, M.D., Robert, J. *The Nazi Doctors*, (New York, Basic Books, 1987) P. 430.

killings.[66] This psychodynamic is exceedingly dangerous for medical professionals because this second self has no moral restraint, and is capable of doing virtually anything. Because this psychological process is so dangerous for society as a whole, euthanasia should not be legalized or tolerated for any reason.

Turning physicians into killers would create not only grave personal problems for health care providers but also grave social consequences as well, as the trustworthiness of the medical profession would be undermined. The ABC television program *Nightline* reported that there were signs that some of the elderly in Holland were reluctant to enter Dutch hospitals because they mistrusted the physicians.[67] For the well-being of all in our anonymous society, it is absolutely necessary to keep our healers from becoming random killers.

Health care providers would find their roles unduly complicated by legalization of mercy killing. Giving them "the killing option" would confront them with the awful question of when they would have to abandon healing and start killing. Without legalized mercy killing, they would not have to confront this option which would be preferable to most health care professionals today. This is the sort of decision that many physicians would consider to be wholly foreign to their professional objectives.

## 4
## The Paradoxes of "Aid-in-Dying"

Besides the practical problems, there are also logical problems in legalized mercy killing. One of the serious problems with "aid-in-dying" is that most of its proponents want the law to permit it to be given quickly so that a person will not have to suffer pain or loss of "dignity" for a long period of time.[68] But the more expeditiously mercy killing is given, the fewer will be the legal

---

[66] *Ibid.* Pp. 416-465.

[67] This criterion for giving euthanasia was explicitly asserted by Dr. Pieter Admiraal in his *Nightline* appearance on February 3, 1987.

[68] See: Mayo, David, Ed. "Contemporary Philosophical Literature on Suicide: A Review", in *Suicide and Ethics*. (New York: Human Sciences Press, 1983)

safeguards to prevent it from being given without warrant to those who do not wish it. Proponents of "aid-in-dying" want to have it both ways: they want to have euthanasia administered in a way that protects individuals from unwanted killing, but they also want it administered so swiftly that "deliverance" from suffering or "indignity" would not be delayed even momentarily. In practice, it is not possible to give mercy killing swiftly to relieve intolerable pain while also giving it only to the rational and in such a way that only those who truly want it are given mercy killing.

A further paradox with legalized "aid-in-dying" is that there is no consensus among suicidologists, physiciatrists, ethicists, philosophers and physicians that choices to end one's life are free and rational.[69] If a patient is truly in a condition of intolerable and untreatable pain, then the freedom of such a person is probably very limited. A choice of such a person would be questionably free because of the limited options available to the person, and also because of the clouded judgment that the person would probably experience from the pain. And if the person did not suffer from intolerable and untreatable pain, there would be a serious question as to whether a choice for death would be in the best interests of the person.

The same can be said of persons who attempt to justify suicide because of a purported loss of dignity. If they have truly lost so much of their dignity that they judge their lives to no longer be worth living, one would have to wonder if they would have sufficient rational power or freedom left to make such a monumental decision. And if they have not lost this dignity, one wonders what good purpose would be served by their choice of death. Mercy killing should not be legalized because it is immoral, and it should certainly not be legalized until the profound difficulties and paradoxes concerning its rationality and freedom have been resolved to the satisfaction of society.

Finally, mercy killing is imprudent because it cannot be done either openly or in secret. If it is done secretly, the possibilities of abuse are so great that it could not be permitted, and there would have to be public scrutiny in order to prevent unwarranted mercy killings. But if this would be done in public it would influence the

---

[69] See: Mayo, D. "Contemporary Philosophical Literature on Suicide: A Review".

immature and unstable to take their own lives. There is thus no possible circumstance in which mercy killing can be practiced in which others could not be positively harmed by it.

Some appear confident that "aid-in-dying" could be legalized in this country with no harmful side effects or consequences. This is not clear either to euthanasia advocates or opponents. In a remarkable series of articles in the *Los Angeles Times* leading proponents of mercy killing admitted they were somewhat frightened about legalization of mercy killing in Holland. Dr. Pieter Admiraal contended that euthanasia for some neurotics or psychotics--even patients with a history of a serious suicide attempt--could be legalized.[70] About that Baroness Adrienne Van Till, herself an advocate of euthanasia, said that "If you make a law that somebody can get help to die simply because he is lonely or psychotic, then that, of course is quite uncontrollable". In the very short run," she said bluntly, "there would be a hell of a lot of abuse."[71] Jean Tromp Meesters, an official of the Dutch Association for Voluntary Euthanasia, even admitted the following about legalized voluntary mercy killing: "I believe [the possibility of eventual societal pressure to accept euthanasia] is very real, and I am very scared about that. "I fear that it is too early for really liberal euthanasia law and it might be too early always."[72]

Others in Holland think that mercy killing is out of control too. Dr. K.F. Gunning, President of the World Federation of Doctors Who Respect Life, conducted a conference on April 26, 1987 and he pointed out that the Dutch *Continuous Morbidity Registration* noted that in 1986 only 3000 patients requested euthanasia. But the most common estimates are that from 6,000 to 18,000 mercy killings were performed in Holland during that year. Thus, he suggests that for every voluntary mercy killing in Holland there were at least one and possibly five involuntary mercy killings.[73] Support for this was

---

[70] "The Netherlands Debates the Legal Limits of Euthanasia", by Allan Parachini. *The Los Angeles Times*, June 5, 1987. Part VI. P. 8, cols. 1-2.

[71] *Ibid.*

[72] *Ibid.*

[73] K.F. Gunning, "Euthanasia in the Netherlands", Unpublished Manuscript. P. 1.

offered in a letter to the *Wall Street Journal* on September 29, 1987 by Dr. Richard Fenigsen, M.D. of the Willem-Alexander Hospital in Hertogenbosch, Netherlands. Dr. Fengisen claimed that the Dutch Patients Association placed a warning in the press that in many hospitals patients are being killed without their will or knowledge, or the knowledge of their families.[74] The notice warned patients to inquire into every step of treatments given in hospitals and when in doubt to consult experts outside of a hospital. It noted further that the *Standpoint on Euthanasia* proposed by the Dutch Royal Society of Medicine was unanimously rejected by the Committee on Medical Ethics of the European Community.

Fenigsen noted that he and his colleagues C.I.Dessaur, C.J.C. Rutenfrans and K.F. Gunning found that involuntary mercy killing as being widely practiced in Holland.[75] They found widespread support for mercy killing, as 43% of those polled supported it for those who were unconscious with little chance for recovery.[76] A doctor suspected of killing 20 residents of a nursing home pleaded guilty to having killed five and was convicted of three. But a higher court discarded the guilty plea and the physicians was only fined $150,000 in damages.[77]

It should be clear that very harmful consequences would accompany legalization of any form of mercy killing. In all likelihood, these harmful consequences will be seen shortly in Holland, and that nation's experiment with mercy killing should be studied very closely. But even if very dangerous practical consequences are not found in the Dutch experiments, we should be very cautious about taking any measures to endorse it in this country because our legal systems are so different and that might not appear in Holland might very well plague us in America.

There is one thing we should not forget about "aid-in dying". No matter what the motives of the mercy killer might be, mercy

---

[74] "Involuntary Euthanasia In Holland" *The Wall Street Journal*, September 29, 1987, P. 17, cols. 1-2.

[75] *Ibid.*

[76] *Ibid.*

[77] *Ibid.*

killing remains the deliberate killing of innocent, sick, disabled, dying and suffering persons precisely because they are so. There might be good reasons for killing people, but killing sick and despairing innocent persons precisely because they are so is not a good justifying reason. Our culture has espoused the principle that killing innocent persons does not resolve problems, and legalization of "aid-in-dying" might very well be a wholesale abridgement of that principle. It is by no means certain that legalized mercy killing will truly resolve any of the serious social problems that will confront our society as it enters the next century, and it might very well destroy some of the traditions that could help us in solving those problems.

## CHAPTER SIX
## FEEDING THE COMATOSE AND THE COMMON GOOD IN THE CATHOLIC TRADITION

At a recent convention sponsored by the Catholic Health Association in Boston, Laurence J. O'Connell, vice-president for ethics and theology, made the following comments:

> I am concerned that some of those who are legitimately alarmed by the potential abuses associated with the public policy that authorizes the withholding and withdrawing of mechanical means of nutrition and hydration are sometimes publicly misrepresenting the Catholic moral tradition. In other words, in their well-intentioned and perfectly legitimate efforts to avoid the slippery-slope that is the wrongful withholding or withdrawing of nutrition or hydration from vulnerable classes of patients these advocates are placing the Roman Catholic moral tradition itself on the slippery slope.
>
> It is mistaken to say it is the church's teaching that we may never withhold or withdraw artificial nutrition and hydration. It is mistaken to uncritically refer to the removal of medically engineered nutrition in all cases as starvation that is, the willful withholding of nutrition as morally obligatory. It is mistaken to say that the ethical standards of a single Catholic hospital are necessarily coextensively with the ethical standards of the Catholic Church. Just because an individual Catholic facility, for whatever reason, uniformly refuses to allow the withholding or withdrawing of technological feeding, does not mean that the Church itself disallows such withholdings or withdrawals.[1]

It is not clear how the Catholic moral tradition can be put on the "slippery slope" by opposing certain forms of withdrawal of feeding from specific classes of patients. Dr. O'Connell has misrepresented the thought of most of those who oppose the recent American Medical Association's new opinion which holds that artificially administered nutrition and fluids can be removed from

---

[1] "Church and State Overlap in Ethical Debate", *American Medical News*. February 27,1987. P. 1.

terminally ill patients, even when they are not imminently dying.[2] There are no Catholic moralists who claim that it is always and everywhere morally wrong to withhold or withdraw feeding from patients. However, there are a number of moralists as well as bishops who now hold it to be wrong to withhold or withdraw feeding in those cases where the withholding or withdrawal becomes the fundamental and underlying cause of death.

O'Connell is probably correct in saying that the policies of one hospital do not necessarily determine the moral doctrines of the universal Church, but neither does one national organization such as the Catholic Health Association with only a loose affiliation with the magisterial hierarchy of the Church, necessarily do this either. The debate over the provision of assisted feeding is a debate over whether it is morally legitimate to withdraw feeding such that the primary and fundamental reason why the person dies is because of that withdrawal. It is a debate over whether those with a certain "quality of life" can be permitted to be killed by omission. It questions whether feeding provided by routine nursing measures that can significantly sustain the life is a medical treatment that should be governed by the criteria governing other treatments, or whether it is an aspect of normal care, like protection from exposure or hygienic care that is to be accorded to all patients.

In this chapter, I wish to review the thoughts of some of the classical Catholic moralists to argue that support can be found in their thought for a conservative policy of providing assisted food and fluids. I also wish to show that where they did establish liberal

---

[2] "Withholding or Withdrawing Life Prolonging Medical Treatment" adopted by the Council on Ethical and Judicial Affairs of the American Medical Associations on March 15, 1987. In its pertinent parts, it stated:

> The social commitment of the physician is to sustain life and relieve suffering. Where the performance of one duty conflicts with the other, the choice of the patient, or his family or legal representative if the patient to act in his own behalf, should prevail.
>
> Life prolonging medical treatment includes medication and artificially or technologically supplied respiration, nutrition or hydration. In treating a terminally ill or irreversibly comatose patient, the physician should determine whether the benefits of treatment outweigh its burdens. At all times, the dignity of the patient should be maintained.

policies for removing assisted food and fluids, their arguments for doing so were flawed and open to severe criticism. And I will also show that assisted feeding can be imposed on patients in some cases because of the demands of the common good.

# A
## THOMAS AQUINAS

Aquinas did not write any treatise devoted specifically to providing food and fluids, but he did note in his *Super Epistolos S. Pauli* that:

> A man has the obligation to sustain his body, otherwise he would be a killer of himself. . .by precept, therefore, he is bound to nourish his body and likewise we are bound to all the other items without which the body cannot live.[3]

In this passage Aquinas affirms an obligation to take food and fluids because of a general obligation to sustain life, and he asserts that failing to take them could be morally equivalent to self-killing in some cases. He apparently would not say this about medical treatments for he would hold it licit to reject medical treatments in some cases without being a self-killer.[4]

The passage implies that there are more circumstances in which one may licitly reject medical treatments than there are where one could reject food and water. Aquinas vaguely asserts a distinction between nutrition and fluids and medical treatments, and he imposes a stronger obligation to receive food and water than to receive medical treatments. The reason why this stronger obligation exists seems to be that food and water are seen as a means of sustaining life whether the person is sick or not, while medical treatments are therapeutic measures only to be used for those with

---

[3] St. Thomas Aquinas, *Super Epistolos S.Pauli* (Taurini-Romae, Marietti, 1953), II Thess., Lec. II, n. 77. Translation in Cronin, Daniel, *The Moral Law in Regard to the Ordinary and Extraordinary Means of Conserving Life*, (Dissertatio ad Lauream in Facultate Theologica Pontificiae Universitatis Gregorianae, Romae,1958) P. 48.

[4] Medical treatments that could be rejected without being a self-killer would be those which are rejected out of a due love for life and for the spiritual goods.

clinical conditions.

In a statement that should be balanced against the previous one, he says in the *Secunda Secundae* that:

> [I]t is inbred for a man to love his own life and those things which contribute to it, but in due measure (*tamen debito proprio*) which means those things which permit attainment of the final goal. Thus, those things which permit attainment of the final end of man are to be loved, but only in due measure.[5]

In the statement prior to this one Aquinas warned against self killing and a lack of respect for life, but in this one he warns against anxious concern for life and undue love for life-preserving measures. This statement imposes an obligation to have due respect for life and to have a moderate love for those things which sustain life. There is a duty to protect one's life by moderate means and he denounces an overly-exaggerated fear of death which can cause an undue clinging to life.

What precisely "due love of the things that sustain life" would be is not clear from this passage. It would seem that Aquinas is objecting to demands for radically expensive treatments that would not hold out much prospect of prolonging life or that would only do so at great cost. If this is true, then it would be hard to see how he could object to assisted feeding for a medically stable patient given by routine nursing procedures, for this would not seem to be an uncommon or exotic means of preserving life.

What he might mean by medical treatments that can permit the attainment of the final end of many is also not clear. He may have been referring to those treatments which enabled a person to act rationally and interpersonally. However, that is unlikely because it would imply that there was no duty to give even palliative care to those who suffered emotional or mental disabilities. What Aquinas probably meant was that treatments which could sustain either biological life itself or human life in all its dimensions had to be given because both of these permit attainment of the final end of

---

[5] *Summa Theologica*, Blackfriars Translation, Anthony Ross, O.P., and P.G. Walsh. (New York: McGraw-Hill, 1966) II,II, q. 126, a. 1.

man. If he did not mean that, it would be hard to see how he could have objected that refusal of feeding in some cases or instances was self-killing.

In relation to our contemporary controversy on assisted feeding, his doctrine would affirm the morality of providing and receiving readily available forms of assisted feeding when their denial or refusal would be the fundamental and underlying cause of death of a medically stable patient. It should be recalled that what is "common" is relative to a society, and in our society, assisted feeding administered by routine nursing measures is simply a common mode of providing nutrition, and it should be provided when its withdrawal would cause death.

## B
## FRANCISCO VITORIA

Francisco Vitoria requires patients to take ordinary measures to preserve life, and he explicitly holds that a patient would have to at least use foods commonly employed by persons to conserve their life.[6] Vitoria affirms an obligation to receive food and water when they can be readily provided by a given society. Only the use of ordinary foods, and not exotic dishes, would be morally required, even if this would shorten the life of the patient. In his own way, he affirms an obligation to give and receive only what are customarily and commonly available forms of care and feeding in a society.

He claims that it is one thing to destroy life and another to cease to protect or prolong it.[7] One must never do the former, but he holds that it is not always necessary to do the latter. This formulation, however, is too vague and general to be useful at the

---

[6] F. Vitoria, *Relectiones Theologicae*, (Lugduni, 1587), Relectio IX, de Temp. n. 1, (Trans. in Cronin, *Op. cit*. Pp. 48-49.) Atkinson notes that the obligation to take drugs is less grave than the obligation to take food because food is *per se* ordered to the preservation of life. See his: "Theological History on the Catholic Teaching on Prolonging Life" in *Moral Responsibility in Prolonging Life Decisions*, edited by Donald McCarthy and Albert Moraczewski, O.P. (St. Louis: Pope John Center, 1981) P. 98.

[7] See: Atkinson, "Theological History of Catholic Teaching on Prolonging Life", p. 98.

present time, for failing to protect life in some instances is morally equivalent to destroying it. For example, permitting another to die by withholding protection from exposure is morally equivalent to destroying that person's life. Similarly, failing to sustain another's life by withholding life-sustaining food and water that can be provided by routine and customary means is morally equivalent to failing to protect life.

Nowhere does Vitoria affirm that "common" feeding could be rejected because this would be killing by omission, but unfortunately, he does not explain what constitutes "common" feeding. What makes feeding "common" would seem to be relative to one's culture and technology, but Vitoria offers no explicit opinion on this. He does teach that taking food is not obligatory if great effort is required, and he probably means great effort on the part of the patient.[8] Taking food when great effort would be demanded of the patient would require a radical exercise of the virtue of fortitude, and Vitoria would not impose such a demand as a matter of justice. The term "common" is purely formal, but it must be assumed to mean what is routinely provided to a patient in a given condition; this criterion is highly relative to the means available of providing food and water. And there is no hint in Vitoria's thought that "ordinary" medical customs could be violated.

He discusses the issue of food and water under the aspect of the virtues, and affirms that failing to receive commonly available life-sustaining food and water would be against the virtue of fortitude, and failing to provide it would seem to be against the virtue of justice.[9] Like Aquinas, he imposes a stronger duty to provide food than to provide medical treatments, for he holds that the obligation to take drugs is less serious than is the obligation to take food. In order for medical treatments to be morally required in some circumstances, it would only be necessary for there to be some hope of returning to normal functioning or some form of recovery. But "common" food and water, or that by which regularly

---

[8] *Ibid.*

[9] *Ibid.* P. 97. Vitoria discusses the taking of food under the aspect of temperance, but it would seem that denial of life-sustaining food and drink to an individual would not be against temperance as much as it would be against justice, while the refusal of life-sustaining food and water would be against the virtue of fortitude.

a man can live (*satis est, quod det operam, per quam homo regulariter potest vivere*), have to be given even if recovery is not possible, but if there is some hope of life.[10] And he makes no explicit distinctions between biological, psychological, and spiritual life, and this implies that food and water must be given if there is some hope of continuing biological or physical life. If there is moral certitude that food and water could hold out "some hope of life" being continued, then it would seem that he would hold it obligatory to provide nutrition and hydration.

For Vitoria, it is not necessary to use every means available to sustain life, but only to use those means which are of themselves intended for that purpose and which are congruent with that end.[11] And if there is a "kind of impossibility in receiving food and water, Vitoria would not require their provision or acceptance. Thus, if there was profound revulsion to food, or a medical reason for rejecting it, he would not morally require it. It is not clear what he means by this, for food and water, hygiene and medicine all naturally aim at preserving life. On this point, Vitoria is ambivalent, for while he admits that food, water and medical treatments are naturally ordered toward life, he affirms a more stringent obligation to provide food and water than to provide medical treatments which would imply that they are different in nature.[12] There is no obligation to use the most expensive and costly treatments or foods to sustain life, but this should not be interpreted to mean that a person could be morally required to suffer destitution to pay for common feeding or ordinary medical

---

[10] *Ibid*. Pp. 98-9. The failure to preserve one's life would be rejection of those things "by which regularly a man can live". This would seem to consist in food and fluids taken orally or what modern authors call "ordinary" surgeries and medical treatments. The modern criterion seems to be that of requiring not just food and fluids but ordinary surgeries as well.

[11] See Atkinson, "Theological History of Catholic Teaching on Prolonging Life", p. 99.

[12] *Relectiones*, Relectio X, de Homicidio, n. 35, (Transl. as in Cronin, p. 50.)

care.[13]

This ambivalence in Vitoria's thought is important, for Fr. Edward Bayer, a contemporary moral theologian, contends that there is an obligation to provide food and water orally or "connaturally", but that obligation ceases when a person needs assisted feeding.[14] For Bayer, the natural aspect of oral feeding imposes the obligation, but it is by no means clear that such a distinction was seen by Vitoria.[15] It is not clear that Vitoria sees the mode of provision as being as crucial as the commonness of the mode of feeding. What is clear with Vitoria's thought, however, is that he believes that the provision of commonly available, life-sustaining food and water is ethically obligatory.

Relative to the contemporary debate on feeding medically stable comatose patients, Vitoria's teachings would imply that assisted feeding and fluids provided as an aspect of basic patient maintenance, could not be withheld from comatose patients because they are now an aspect of "common" feeding. He would not require their provision if it was medically impossible to provide them, or if the person was unable to receive them for clear medical reasons, and he does not demand that radical or extreme expense be experienced to provide them. But if receiving or providing food or water is "common" in a given culture, he would hold it to be morally required. He considered food and water to be different in nature from medical treatments, and he established different criteria for their provision and acceptance. He admits that there are elective forms of feeding, but those that are common modes of feeding are morally mandatory. By asserting that there is a stronger obligation to take food than there is to take medical treatments, he is affirming the principle that if assisted feeding and fluids provided as an aspect of basic patient maintenance could meet the nutritional

---

[13] *Ibid.* P. 99. He affirms that expensive or exotic foods would not be required, and he does not hold that one would have to live in the most healthful climates either. See his: *Commentaria a la Secunda Secundae de Santo Thomas*, (Salamanca, ed. de Hereda, O.P., 1952) in II-II, q. 147, a (Transl. as in Cronin, p. 59).

[14] *Ibid.*

[15] "Foregoing Life-Sustaining Food and Water: 1900 Years of Catholic Thought". Unpublished Manuscript. Pp. 1-2.

# MEDICAL ETHICS

and hydrational needs of the patient, they should be given.

## C
## JUAN CARDINAL DE LUGO

In the century after Vitoria, there was widespread support among moral theologians for his teachings. Juan Cardinal de Lugo is important because he supported Vitoria's teachings, but also because he drew clearer distinctions between morally permissible letting-die and immoral killing based on the type of means being refused or withheld. He is noteworthy for being exceptionally liberal among his contemporaries for his view of what constituted an extraordinary means.[16] Because of this, Atkinson notes that he was so liberal in his views that he accepted virtually any reason whatsoever for removing a medical treatment. For instance, he held that drinking wine or abstaining from it could be an extraordinary form of care in some cases.

With regard to the administration of extraordinary treatments, De Lugo claims that a person caught in a burning building would not have to use water to extinguish part of the fire, thus only delaying momentarily the time of death, because partially extinguishing the fire would be a futile attempt to preserve life.[17] This example is strictly applicable to a patient who is truly dying and for whom assisted feeding would not substantially sustain life. In such a case, the removal of food and fluids would not be the underlying and fundamental cause of death as would be the fire, and it would therefore be permissible to remove them.

But whether these sorts of patients would have to be fed is not the issue today. The pertinent issue is whether the removal of feeding should be morally permitted when its removal would be the fundamental cause of death. He holds that the only condition necessary for providing food and water is that there be "some hope

---

[16] Atkinson, "Theological History of Catholic Teachings on Prolonging Life", pp. 101-2.

[17] De Lugo, Juan. *Disputationes Scholasticae et Morales*, (ed. nova, Parisiis, Vives, 1868-69), Vol. VI, *De Justitia et Jure*, Disp. X, Sec. 1, n. 21. (Transl. as in Cronin, p. 59).

of sustaining life".[18] The term "some" does not mean that it be absolutely certain that life will be sustained, but only that there be some prospect of it being continued by the provision of food and water. This requirement that feeding be given when there is some hope of life being preserved would seem to require its provision in that case.

He is one of the few classical moralists to give high priority to the judgment of a physician, and if a competent and upright physician determines that a treatment is necessary he would require the patient to consent to the treatment.[19] De Lugo was primarily concerned with the morality of mutilations, and he held that they were obligatory if they could cure and if they did not involve great pain. If a mutilating therapy would be necessary for the health or well-being of the patient, but the patient rejected it, De Lugo would compel its acceptance.[20] De Lugo states that a patient:

> must permit [a] cure when the doctors judge it necessary, and when it can happen without intense pain; not, if it is accompanied by very bitter pain; because a man is not bound to employ extraordinary and difficult means to conserve life.[21]

According to De Lugo, the failure to employ reasonably available means of preserving life could be equivalent to taking one's life, but he does not identify the conditions under which this might occur.[22] This principle applies when the means are not difficult to use and when death from the lethal cause could be easily

---

[18] Atkinson, "Theological History of Catholic Teachings on Prolonging Life", p. 102.

[19] De Lugo, *loc. cit.*

[20] It is likely that De Lugo held this to prevent patients from committing suicide by rejecting medically indicated, beneficial and nonburdensome treatments from being provided.

[21] J. De Lugo, *Disputationes Scholasticae et Morales*, Vol, VI, *De Justitia et Jure*, Disp. X, Sec. 1, n. 21.

[22] Atkinson, "Theological History of Catholic Teaching on Prolonging Life", p. 102.

avoided. This would imply that assisted feeding would be required if it was readily available and if its provision could prevent death by starvation or dehydration. Thus, De Lugo was deeply concerned about the morality of removing food and water from patients, and he clearly believed that some withdrawals were immoral.

## D
## GERALD KELLY, S, J.

### a
### The Usefulness of Assisted Feeding

Fr. Gerald Kelly is important in the history of contemporary Catholic medical ethics because of his development of the doctrine of ordinary and extraordinary means. He developed his views on the requirements to receive medical treatments, and in his later writings he established a clearer normative position on the duties to receive care and treatment. Kelly claims that families and medical professionals should be brought into treatment decisions because they have moral duties demanding respect.[23] In holding this, he laid a foundation for the contemporary "covenental" theory of medical decisionmaking espoused by Paul Ramsey.[24]

In this advanced views, Kelly provides us with the what has come to be accepted as the "classical" definition of ordinary and extraordinary means:

> *Ordinary* means are all medicines, treatments and operations which offer a reasonable hope of benefit and which can be obtained and used without excessive expense, pain or other inconvenience.
>
> *Extraordinary* means are all medicines, treatments and

---

[23] *Ibid*. P . 107. Kelly mentions this, it seems, to affirm that families and health care providers have duties to provide care and that authorization of withdrawal of care by either of these can constitute culpable killing.

[24] See: Paul Ramsey, *The Patient as Person*, (Princeton: Princeton University Press, 1979) and *Basic Christian Ethics*, (Chicago: University of Chicago Press, 1950. Pp. 367-388.

operations which cannot be obtained and used without excessive expense, pain or other inconvenience, or which if used, would not offer a reasonable hope of benefit.[25]

After making this distinction, he proceeds to ask if there could be a "useless ordinary" means of preserving life and if such a means could be morally required. Initially, Kelly argues that all ordinary means are obligatory, but this changes in his later works and replies that no one can be required to employ a means that is useless. He therefore declared some ordinary means to be elective because they were "useless".[26] He writes:

> [N]o *remedy* is obligatory unless it offers *a reasonable hope of checking or curing the disease*. I would not call this a common opinion because many authors do not refer to it, but I know of no one who opposes it, and it seems to have intrinsic merit as an application of the axiom, *nemo ad inutile tenetur* [i.e., No one can be obliged to do what is useless]. Moreover, it squares with the rule commonly applied to the analogous case of helping one's neighbor: one is not obliged to offer help unless there is a reasonable assurance that it will be efficacious.[27]

Kelly argues correctly that a treatment is useless if it does not offer a reasonable hope of checking or curing a disease. In light of this definition, it would seem that provision of food and fluids by assisted means would be useful when it could prevent the person from succumbing from starvation or dehydration. For in that circumstance, it could "check" the "disease" of starvation.

Oddly, Kelly argues that there would be no obligation to provide fluids and feeding to a patient by assisted means if the patient was unconscious and was expected to die within a few

---

[25] G. Kelly, "The Duty to Preserve Life", *Theological Studies*, XII, (1951) P. 550.

[26] G. Kelly, "The Duty of Using Artificial Means of Preserving Life" *Theological Studies*, XI, (1950), pp. 218-9.

[27] *Ibid.* Pp. 207-8.

weeks.[28] In this situation food and water should be provided because they could achieve their end of preventing death from death by dehydration or starvation and thus would not be useless because they could "check the disease". Kelly does not hold that life-sustaining measures would have to "check disease for a certain period of time", but only that they have this power. It is thus peculiar that Kelly considers assisted feeding useless simply because its power is temporally limited.

Further application of his principle would imply that feeding which could only sustain life for short period of time is "useless" would also seem to allow spoon-feeding to be withdrawn or withheld from a conscious terminally ill patient with even more time to live, because spoon-feeding is more burdensome to others than is tube feeding. It could permit withholding insulin from a diabetic who was expected to live for a couple of weeks, even though its withdrawal would cause death, and it might even permit withdrawal of hygienic care or protection from exposure. Kelly's understanding of utility is correct but it seems that he did not apply it properly in practice, for he did not see that feeding could fend off death for a limited period of time and was therefore useful. He is correct in saying that useless treatments need not be given, but he fails to see that some forms of assisted feeding were not useless when they could prevent death from dehydration or starvation even for a limited period of time by their mere provision.

Kelly's belief that there should be no obligation to continue feeding a patient expected to die within two weeks if the patient is unconscious is quite remarkable. He asserts that a conscious patient should be permitted to decide whether or not to receive feeding, but he holds there is no duty to give food and water to one in a similar state but unconscious.[29] This view would radically limit the obligations of health care providers to the unconscious terminal patient, and it implies the moral permissibility of abandoning provision of all treatment for them. It is also quite discriminatory because it implies that capacity for psychological relating is the ground for the possession of moral rights. Kelly would undoubtedly

---

[28] *Ibid.* P. 220.

[29] *Ibid.* P. 219.

object to recently enacted Baby Doe Regulations of the Child Abuse Act which prohibited the removal of food and water from comatose infants, despite the fact that strong approval was given these regulations by the disabled community.[30]

Kelly's argument in favor of removing feeding from unconscious terminally ill patients is pertinent to the contemporary issue of providing feeding for the medically stable comatose. For, under some definitions of euthanasia, withdrawing food and water from them would be mercy killing because the withdrawal would be done for the purpose of causing death to prevent a patient from experiencing severe pain.[31] Kelly correctly argued that the removal of some medical treatments in such cases was permissible, but feeding should not be withdrawn because doing so would cause death as surely as would a lethal injection.

The withdrawal of food and water, provided as an aspect of normal patient maintenance or routine nursing care is not merely the "occasion" of the patient's death, but is its cause.[32] When one removes or refrains from throwing a life ring to a man who would drown without it, the removal or withholding is not the "occasion" of the man's death but is the cause. Similarly, the removal or withholding of these readily providable forms of feeding is the causes of the death of a patient who would be medically stable with their provision. He allows this withdrawal even though it would imply that death could be physically caused by removing a routinely available means of preserving life. Kelly ignores the issue of causation of death, and he seems to feel that there would be nothing

---

[30] *Nondiscrimination on the Basis of Handicap; Procedures and Guidelines Relating to Health Care for Handicapped Infants*, 49 Fed. Reg. 1622, 1623 (January 1983). HHS reported that after a period of comment, 16,739 comments were received, 98.5% of which were favorable. See: "The Emergence of Institutional Ethics Committees" by Ronald E. Cranford and A. Edward Doudera, in their *Institutional Ethics Committees and Health Care Decisions*, (Ann Arbor: Health Administration Press, 1984) P. 5

[31] Webster's Dictionary defines it as an "act or method of causing death painlessly, so as to end suffering" *Webster's New World Dictionary* (Second College Edition) ed. David B. Guralnik (Englewood Cliffs, N.J: Prentice Hall, 1970) P. 889.

[32] The claim that withdrawal of life-sustaining nutrition and fluids that are readily providable does not kill the patient, but is merely the occasion on which the patient succumbs. See: *The Medical-Moral Newsletter*, Vol. 24, No. 4, April 1987, P. 3.

wrong with causing death if death was expected in only a matter of days.

Kelly's endorsement of withdrawing feeding from a comatose patient who was expected to die shortly did not go uncontested, however, for Fr. Joseph Donovan argued that IV feeding was an ordinary medical treatment and that there was no impossibility in feeding the comatose.[33] He claimed that removing feeding in situations where Kelly permitted it was morally equivalent to causing death, and he essentially charged Kelly with endorsing mercy killing by omission when death was imminent.[34]

Kelly agreed that tube feeding was an ordinary medical treatment and he justified this position by making assertions that many would question today. For example, he claimed that this form of feeding was an ordinary medical treatment in the speculative order but that it was an extraordinary treatment in the practical order because it was clinically useless.[35] By admitting that assisted feeding was speculatively obligatory but practically elective, Kelly implicitly affirmed that there were aspects of assisted feeding that differentiated it from other forms of therapeutic, palliative or remedial medical treatment. But Kelly was unable to see this difference precisely, and he did not impose obligations correlative to this difference. Kelly would have had no trouble teaching that a therapeutic procedure such as an appendectomy for a dying person was useless because the person would die from the other cause before he or she died from the appendicitis, and he seemed to think that assisted feeding could become extraordinary in exactly the same sense. What he did not see, however, was that withdrawing successful and readily providable feeding creates a new and independent lethal condition, irrespective of the clinical picture of the patient.

The inconsistency of Kelly's thought compromises his claims about the optional character of assisted feeding for various classes

---

[33] Fr. Donovan's article appeared in *Homiletic and Pastoral Review*, XLIX, (August, 1949) P. 72

[34] Kelly, G. "The Duty of Using Artificial Means of Preserving Life", P. 210.

[35] Atkinson, G. "Theological History of Catholic Teaching on Prolonging Life", P. 109.

of patients. Kelly's view that care and treatment can be speculatively ordinary, but practically elective, is not tenable today, and his authority on the issue can be rightfully challenged. His distinction between the speculative and practical has never been widely accepted by medical ethicists, and it is of uncertain utility. It is interesting that Kelly's argument for withdrawing food and fluids was never accepted into the mainstream of Catholic ethical teaching, even though his conclusion was. And conversely, Donovan's arguments were logically sound and implanted in the tradition, but they have been rejected in recent decades.

Kelly also failed to face the issue of causality squarely, for the withdrawal of feeding from such a person was not the mere occasion of death but was in fact the cause of death. It seems that Donovan was correct and that Kelly did in fact permit those near death to be killed by dehydration and starvation. Some contemporary right-to-die activists have charged that the Catholic tradition has allowed mercy killing by omission because of Kelly's views, and there seems to be support for this charge.[36]

Kelly was apparently unaware of a difference between ordinary medical treatments and what some ethicists are now calling normal care or minimal care.[37] This category consists of hygienic care, protection from exposure, psychological support, feeding, and the maintenance of such devices as urinary catheters. Some now believe that to withhold these forms of care would be morally equivalent to killing by omission, but Kelly mentions none of this and it is not evident that he had a clear idea of what constituted killing by omission.

### b
### Assisted Feeding and the Common Good

---

[36] See: Larue, G. *Euthanasia and Religion*, (Los Angeles: Hemlock Press, 1981) Kelly himself feared that his views might be interpreted as being "Catholic Euthanasia". See: "The Duty of Using Artificial Means of Preserving Life", P. 219.

[37] See: Smith, W.B. "Judeo-Christian Teaching on Euthanasia: Definitions, Distinctions and Decisions" *The Linacre Quarterly*, February, 1987, Vol. 54, No. 1, P. 29. Also see: Barry, R. "The Ethics of Providing Life-Sustaining Nutrition and Fluids to Incompetent Patients", *The Journal of Family And Culture*, Vol. I, No. 2, Summer, 1985, P. 27.

More positively, Kelly is about the only moralist in the recent Catholic tradition to explicitly state that patients could be required to use extraordinary and *per se* elective measures if these were required by the common good or a higher value.[38] This is a valuable insight, and it should be applied to protecting society from the emergence of socially and legally endorsed mercy killing. The common good can require a person to accept assisted feeding in order to prevent the social and legal endorsement of euthanasia by omission which would pose a clear threat to the handicapped, immature, unstable and medically vulnerable from mercy killing. Kelly holds that a civil leader can be required to receive medical treatments, and that a father of a family could be morally required to receive them to protect his family.[39] If saving one's life was necessary for the welfare of one's family or the security of a nation, it would be necessary to do so.[40] A common good exists where there is a common goal, and in the case of society, that goal is the well-being of all, and not just the maximization of individual liberties or rights.[41] The good of the community is prior to private interest, and the individual is duty bound to strive for the common good.

The common good can place demands on individuals, but there are limits to what it can require. First, nowhere is an individual released from the duty to do what is morally good, and appeals to the common good cannot release one from this

---

[38] Kelly, G. "The Duty of Using Artificial Means of Preserving Life", P. 206.

[39] *Ibid*. P. 216.

[40] See: Welty, Eberhard, *Handbook of Christian Social Ethics*. (New York: Herder & Herder: 1963). P. 312.

[41] St. Thomas says that "[T]he community has necessarily the same goal as the individual." "The good of the individual is not a final end but is subordinated to the common good." "Individual well-being cannot exist without the welfare of the community. . .therefore it is judging correctly in the light of the common good that man must recognize what is good for him." *Summa Theologica*, II-II 58, 6-7. See: Welty. *op. cit.* P. 94. This principle is in harmony with what some moralists call "universal justice" for such demands to be made. Universal justice is the most important of the natural virtues, according to Thomas.

obligation.[42] Second, the order of values must be preserved which means that higher values must be protected at the expense of lower ones.[43] Thus, morality can be promoted at the expense of art or economic interest, for example. Third, in times of grave crisis, higher values can be set aside for the attainment of lower ones.[44] For example, educational activities can be suspended in time of war for the welfare of the entire community. Extraordinary measures can be commanded for the common good, such that a person can be required to make personal sacrifices to save another's life if that can be done without putting one's self or family in the same danger. Thus, one can be required to forego certain material advantages to protect the lives of others.

Acting in behalf of the common good is required by justice, and is commanded by the virtue of universal justice which seeks to protect the well being of all by directing all actions toward the common good.[45] The virtue of universal justice determines what demands can be imposed on a community by the common good. Virtues can be required by universal justice so that courage could be required in war, just as temperance could be commanded in times of famine.[46] Requiring that extraordinary forms of care or treatment be imposed by the common good is in accord with the principles of universal justice because it is an act of courage for the benefit of the entire community. They can be set aside in specific circumstances so that the individual can pursue the common good.

Assisted feeding could be legally and morally mandated for certain classes because allowing them to reject it or be denied it would place entire classes of handicapped, despairing, terminal and chronically sick patients at risk. Because there is so much imprecision in medical diagnosis and prognosis, feeding should be required for all where it is medically possible so that those who

[42] Welty, *Handbook of Christian Social Ethics.* P. 112.

[43] *Ibid.* Pp. 112-3.

[44] *Ibid.* Pp. 113.

[45] *Ibid.* P. 312-313.

[46] *Ibid.* Pp. 32-3.

should be justly given feeding are not denied it.

By way of summary, one must be careful about invoking Kelly uncritically on the issue of assisted feeding, for there were evident weaknesses in his thought. To his credit, he admits that his principles were inherently imprecise, and he argues that if one is to err in ambiguous situations, it should be on the side of life. He gave us many of the fundamental concepts by which we understand medical ethics today, but some of his analyses were not adequately consistent or insightful. He apparently did not believe that it was possible to kill terminally ill patients by denial of assisted feeding, and he gave no evidence of medically stable but comatose patients or persons with disabilities wishing to end their lives by starvation or dehydration, and thus he is in some respects not the surest of guides for today's problems. Some of his contemporaries such as Fr. Donovan saw this and were critical of his insights, but Donovan's thought has not been given the prominent place that was given to Kelly's in Catholic medical-ethical tradition. This rebuts claims that the moral doctrines of the Church should not be conditioned by public policy considerations, for Kelly explicitly asserts that the moral teachings of the Church do take into consideration issue of public policy.

## E
## DANIEL CRONIN

Daniel Cronin teaches that ordinary means hold out a hope of beneficial results, are commonly used, are proportionate to one's social position, and are not difficult to employ. Even though he does not say when it would actually become so, he agrees that even feeding could become extraordinary if it was useless.[47] It could also be rejected if it was impossible to provide, required great effort to receive, caused great pain, was radically expensive, or caused intense revulsion.[48] For Cronin, the patient possesses the dominant right to decide what treatments are ordinary or extraordinary, and if the

---

[47] Atkinson, "Theological History of Catholic Teaching on Prolonging Life", pp. 110-111.

[48] *Ibid.*

patient is incompetent, the physician should provide only ordinary treatments.[49] Cronin demands that the physician not only avoid practicing euthanasia, but also avoid even giving the impression of practicing it.

Commenting on Vitoria's views on feeding patients, Cronin says the following:

> food is primarily intended by nature for the basic sustenance of animal life. Food for man is basically and fundamentally necessary from the very beginning of his temporal existence. It is basically required by this human life and nature intends food for this for this purpose. That is why man has the right to grow food and kill animals. Furthermore, because it is a law of nature that man sustain himself by food, it is a duty for man to nourish himself by food. In the case of drugs and medicines, the same is not true. Drugs and medicines are intended *per se* by nature to help man conserve his life. However, this is not by way of exception. Drugs and medicines are not the basic way by which man is to nourish his life. They are intended by nature to aid man in the conservation of his life when he is sick or in pain or unable to sustain himself by natural means. These artificial means are not natural means but they are intended by nature to help man protect, sustain and conserve his life. If man were never to be sick, he would never need medicines. If he is sick, however, it is quite *natural* for him to make use of *artificial* means of *conserving life*.[50]

It is hard to see how these conditions, would make assisted feeding optional for the comatose patient because these patients apparently do not experience pain, and tube feeding is apparently less burdensome for others than is spoon feeding. Thus, it would seem permissible to conclude that Cronin would not permit assisted feeding and fluids to be withdrawn from a patient if so doing would be the fundamental cause of death.

---

[49] *Ibid.* Pp. 112-113.

[50] *Ibid.* Pp. 113-114.

# F
# JOSEPH SULLIVAN

Joseph Sullivan acknowledges that there is a difference between feeding and medical treatments.[51] He argues that ordinary means of preserving life are required of all patients, but he does affirm that there are two kinds of ordinary treatments. On the one hand, there are artificial ordinary treatments, such as surgeries, X-rays, transfusions and IV feedings.[52] On the other hand, he suggests that there are natural ordinary means of preserving life such as feeding, protection from exposure, exercise and regular diet.[53] He argues that a natural means of prolong life is *per se* ordinary and yet it could become *per accidens* extraordinary.[54]

Sullivan argues that a cancer patient in extreme pain with

---

[51] Joseph V. Sullivan, *Catholic Teaching on the Morality of Euthanasia*, (Washington: Catholic University of America Press, 1949) Pp. 65.

[52] Sullivan asserts:

> As artificial means, we may understand such means as major and minor operations, x-ray treatments, blood transfusions, intravenous feeding, radium treatments, psychotherapy, oxygen tents, iron lungs, all germicides and antiseptics and even the taking of prepared medicines. *Ibid.* P. 65.

One would wonder if Sullivan would allow withdrawal of antiseptics if it was judged they were too burdensome or useless for the patient. This is asked because many would consider such forms of care as antiseptics as simply normal care, like intravenous feeding, and not artificial medical treatments.

[53] Sullivan holds that the following are natural ordinary means of preserving life:

> Among the natural means of preserving life would be included such means as proper clothing, housing, physical recreation, good food, regularity at meals, etc. *Ibid.* P. 65.

[54] He writes that:

> A natural means of prolonging life is, per se, an ordinary means of prolonging life, yet per accidens may be extraordinary...An artificial means of prolonging life may be an ordinary means or an extraordinary means relative to the physical condition of the patient. *Ibid.* P. 65.

a toleration for painkillers could have food and water removed, even if the patient could live a good while because of a strong heart:

> 1. A cancer patient is in extreme pain and his system has gradually established what physicians call a "toleration" of any drug, so that increased doses give only brief respite from the ever-recurring pain. The attending physician knows that the disease is incurable and that the person is slowly dying, but because of a good heart, it is possible that the agony will continue for several weeks. The physician then remembers that there is one thing that he can do to end the suffering. He can cut off intravenous feeding and the patient will surely die. He does this and before the next day the patient is dead.

> 2. The case involves the principle that an ordinary means of prolonging life and an extraordinary means are relative to the patient's physical condition. Intravenous feeding is an artificial means of prolonging life and therefore one may be more liberal in application of principle. Since this cancer patient is beyond all hope of recovery and suffering extreme pain, intravenous feeding should be considered an extraordinary means of prolonging life. The physician was justified in stopping the intravenous feeding.[55]

These views can be challenged because it is clear that the intention of withholding the food and water is to cause death in order to end suffering.[56] We should recall that euthanasia is "an act or method of causing death painlessly so as to end suffering", and the explicit purpose of removing feeding is not to remove a treatment which itself causes great pain to the patient, but to cause death so that suffering from the disease will cease. If the means of

---

[55] *Ibid.* P. 73.

[56] How one can withdraw readily providable assisted feeding from a medically stable patient without intending death is not clear. Death is as certain as if it were caused by a lethal injection, and death is not a side effect of an act eliminating suffering, but the means by which the suffering was eliminated.

delivering the feeding were the cause of the patient's pain, it might be justified to withdraw it. It is not clear how what he endorses is distinguished from mercy killing by omission.

It is interesting that Sullivan mentions nothing of Kelly's claim that even extraordinary means can be forced on a patient for the common good. And he does not discuss Vitoria's or de Lugo's claim that feeding should be given when there is "some hope of life". They saw not only a difference between feeding and other forms of medical treatment, but they also affirmed that different sorts of criteria governed their provision. Sullivan saw none of this, and simply affirmed that the same criteria governed the provision of food and water in all circumstances. He did not discuss the issue of causality of providing feeding, and he did not say why the failure to provide or receive naturally or artificially ordinary means was immoral. Had he done this, he might have been more willing to establish a stricter criterion for the provision of natural and assisted feeding.

## G
## CHARLES McFADDEN

Charles McFadden believes that the temporary use of medical treatments, including assisted feeding and hydration, is ordinary while their long-term use would be extraordinary.[57] This

---

[57] McFadden writes:

> Routine medical practice today utilizes intravenous feeding in a countless variety of cases. Certainly the physician regards this procedure as an *ordinary* means of conserving life. It is obviously able to be carried out, under normal hospital conditions, without any notable inconvenience. For this reason, we must regard recourse to intravenous feeding, in the case of typical hospitalized patients, as an *ordinary* and morally compulsory procedure.
>
> The above conclusion applies, as stated, to routine hospital cases where the procedure is envisioned as a *temporary* means of carrying a patient through a critical period. Surely any effort to sustain life *permanently* in this fashion would constitute a grave hardship and not be morally compulsory. [Charles J. McFadden, *The Dignity of Life*, (Huntington, Ind.: Our Sunday Visitor Press, 1976). P. 152.]

One must question this judgment. Intravenous feeding is less burdensome than giving

view is questionable because it would seem to imply that the long term use of insulin by a diabetic or spoon feeding of the senile would also be an extraordinary treatment as well. The difficulty is that it is no more burdensome to give assisted feeding than to give spoon feeding, and declaring assisted feeding useless would strongly imply that the long-term use of more burdensome forms of care or treatment such as wheelchairs, or even visual aids for the visually impaired would be extraordinary. McFadden was apparently seeking to be compassionate to the terminal by articulating this principle, but in so doing he created a principle that could place many medically vulnerable persons in jeopardy.

## CONCLUSION

In light of these findings, it does not seem possible to hold that the Catholic medical ethical tradition would be subverted by asserting that feeding be provided when it is an aspect of basic patient maintenance. It cannot simply be said that without qualification the "tradition" permitted assisted feeding and fluids to be removed. It does not appear true that the Catholic tradition simply allowed feeding to be withdrawn from patients because the majority of these writers prohibited the withdrawal of feeding when it was an aspect of basic patient maintenance.

This does not appear to be true for three reasons. First, many in the tradition asserted principles that would not allow removal of life-sustaining food and water from patients, and many in the tradition who argued for its removal failed to provide adequate reasons for that judgment. Second, a number of recent official teachings on this issue have affirmed obligations to feed. And third, there is an emerging consensus within the Church that this sort of feeding is morally necessary. The Catholic social justice tradition affirms duties of justice to give food and drink to those in need.

Thus, Aquinas would not permit self-killing, and he required

---

some Alzheimer's patients spoon feeding. Does that mean that feeding those patients permanently would also be elective and not obligatory? Would the permanent use of colostomies also be elective if they were required for long term use? Many individuals now live with the aid of portable respirators. Are those elective also, despite the fact that people can lead largely normal lives with them?

that commonly available feeding be provided and accepted by all persons. Vitoria demanded that feeding be given as long as there was "some hope of life". De Lugo, despite his laxity on many issues, affirmed that feeding be given and received as long as there was "some hope of life", and he held that the refusal of reasonably available means to sustain life would be morally equivalent to suicide.

Gerald Kelly demanded that extraordinary treatments to be given when required by the common good, and this would certainly include assisted feeding in some cases. When he did allow life-sustaining, readily available assisted feeding to be withdrawn, he defended that judgment poorly by arguing that feeding was speculatively ordinary but practically extraordinary. Kelly's critics were more consistent in their logic than he was, but they were not given the place in the "tradition" accorded to Kelly. Daniel Cronin admitted a difference between nutrition and fluids and medical treatments, but he did not draw out the implications of this difference. As a result of this he did not see that there should be different criteria governing the provision of food and water than governed the administration of medical treatments.

Joseph Sullivan admitted that there was a difference between feeding and other forms of ordinary care, but he permitted feeding to be removed from a cancer patient who was in great pain but who would live a long while because of a strong heart. But because the intention of the action was to end the life of a person in extreme suffering his view is questionable because it seems to be endorsing euthanasia by omission. He elided natural feeding into the category of ordinary medical treatment by requiring its provision according to the same standards as those governing ordinary medical care. Previous authors asserted stricter obligations to provide ordinary feeding, but Sullivan would not accept this. He recognized that there was a difference between natural and assisted feeding, but he did not see that a different type of obligation should flow from that difference. And Charles McFadden allowed permanent assisted feeding to be removed because it was a burden, but he did not say how this was a burden to the comatose patient, the first individual to be considered in making these estimates.

Second, in the past decade, a number of important official statements have been issued on the provision of food and water to patients, and these have support the view that quality of life judgments are not to be allowed determine if feeding is to be given. The *Declaration on Euthanasia* held that it was legitimate to refrain from using remedies when existence was precarious and painful, but it held that ordinary means had to be provided.[58] In *The Matter of Nancy Ellen Jobes*, the New Jersey Catholic Conference filed an *amicus curiae* brief arguing that this severely brain damaged, but medically stable young woman be fed.[59]

Immediately after the Judicial Council of the American Medical Association issued its opinion that considered removal of food and water from comatose patients who were not imminently dying, Archbishop Philip Hannan condemned the Judicial Council's opinion.[60] And after an appellate court in California ordered caregivers and a hospital to remove a feeding tube which they gave Elizabeth Bouvia because they thought she was trying to starve herself to death, Archbishop Roger Mahony called the decision irrational.[61] Most recently, in the lead editorial in the Jesuit theological journal *La Civita Cattolica*, which is often a mouthpiece for the Vatican's thinking on issues, withholding "ordinary means" such as food, blood transfusions and injections" was rejected as

---

[58] *Declaration on Euthanasia*, Sacred Congregation for the Doctrine of the Faith, May 5, 1980.

[59] Brief, *Amicus Curiae*, and appendix, *In the Matter of Nancy Ellen Jobes*, on Behalf of the New Jersey Catholic Conference, #26, 041. P. 5.

[60] In a letter on March 16, 1986, Archbishop Hannan wrote the following:

> The Catholic Church has always held that families are not obligated to use extraordinary means -- such as artificial life support systems -- to sustain the life of a patient in a hopelessly irreversible coma. However, food and water are ordinary means of sustaining life. Therefore, the Catholic Church opposes the American Medical Association position because it approves denying a person the normal nourishment that he or she needs to sustain life.

[61] "Mahony Critical of Logic in Bouvia Case", *San Fernando Valley Daily News*, April 24, 1986. P. 1. In addition, Cardinals Law and Bernardin also criticized decisions to allow food and water to be removed from patients. See: "Law Takes Side in Coma Case", *The Boston Herald*, June 8, 1985, and "Cardinal Warns of Euthanasia", *Chicago Catholic*, April 16, 1986.

immoral.[62] These statements clearly show that a consensus is emerging in the official teachings of the Church on the moral obligation to provide assisted feeding when it is an aspect of basic patient maintenance. It is clear that through these official statements, the magisterium is correcting what might be deficiencies in the moral theological tradition of recent years and is teaching that withholding life sustaining feeding is killing by omission.

Third, giving food and drink to those in need is in clear harmony with classical Catholic social justice principles. There is an emerging consensus that those who have the financial means and technological capability feed the needy must put their means to that use. This moral perceived obligation motivated recent efforts by Western nations to feed the starving in Africa through *Live Aid*, and major economic, scientific and agricultural efforts to promote the development of agriculture in the third world. This obligation has been repeatedly affirmed in recent Papal Encyclicals which have called on the rich nations to care for those nations which cannot feed themselves, and it is imposed on the rich nations as a matter of justice. The Encyclical *Populorum Progressio* expressed concern for the growing problem of hunger in the world and it saw depressing despondency as a consequence of this hunger.[63]

This issue of providing feeding patients is part and parcel of this problem. Lack of food was viewed as posing hazards greater than were immediately apparent, and it considered lack of food and water an ancient scourge. The Holy Father simply asserted "No

---

[62] *La Civita Cattolica*, February 21, 1987. The editorial cited the report of the Vatican Commission "Cor Unum" which stated:

> There remains the strict obligation to apply under all circumstances those therapeutic measures which are called 'minimal': that is, those which are normally and customarily used for the maintenance of life (food, blood transfusions, injections, etc.)

The editorial also criticized efforts to withhold "ordinary means" of treatment such as food, blood transfusions or injections. See: "Euthanasia Spreading, Jesuit Journal Warns" *The Boston Pilot*, March 6, 1987.

[63] *Populorum Progressio*, Para. 45. See: Joseph Gremillion, *The Gospel of Peace and Justice*, (Maryknoll, N.Y.: Orbis Books, 1979). P. 401.

more hunger, hunger never again!"[64] He did not just say this about the hunger of the poor, but about hunger in general. The Holy Father said that the lack of prudent economic planning was one reason why some suffered hunger.[65] This point should be taken seriously with respect to assisted feeding for many have sought to justify its removal precisely for economic reasons. The Holy Father asserted that the right to satisfy one's hunger must finally be recognized for everyone, according to the specific requirements of his age and activity, and he called for vigilance and courage to feed the hungry.[66]

The obligation to feed the hungry seems to be based on the Gospel story of the Good Samaritan. The failure to give food and drink to the nameless stranger is denounced as not just a failure of charity, but particularly a serious failure in justice. The Samaritan does not stop to investigate the medical condition of the victim of brigands, but simply gives food and drink. Those who fail to do this are not depicted as merely being lacking in charity, but as being hateful and maliciously selfish and egocentric. The Good Samaritan, is really depicted as being more of a "minimally decent" Samaritan who simply does what common decency demand. He does not ask if the man will survive a long period of time, fully recover his capability for human action, or be able to act for human spiritual and affective ends. He does not ask if his actions will increase his sufferings, and he certainly does not "put the man out of his misery" by giving him a "quick and painless death"!

This is general obligation to give food and drink does not cease when nursing techniques are needed to provide them, for it is probably easier to give IV or NG feeding to a hospital patient in the United States than it is a starving person in the African or South American countryside, for instance. Thus, to permit food and water to be withheld from those who can live with its mere provision as a matter of social policy could undermine this developing moral

---

[64] "Address of His Holiness Pope Paul VI to the Participants of the World Food Conference, Rome (Nov. 9, 1974), para. 2. In Gremillion, *op. cit.* Pp. 599-606.

[65] *Ibid.* Para. 2, 3. Pp. 602-606

[66] *Ibid.*

consensus that food must be given by those with the capability to all people.

Food and water, irrespective of their mode of provision, are basic resources of the body, are not therapeutic measures and are matters of basic human rights. They are used by every cell, organ and system in the body to sustain its natural functions, and their natural finality or teleological orientation is not therapeutic. Unlike medical treatments, all people require them whether they are well or ill. To remove them when their mere provision by routine techniques of patient maintenance is to kill the patient by omission through their denial. Removing them does not allow an underlying pathological condition to be set free, but sets the process of dying immediately into motion.

In affirming that life-sustaining assisted feeding provided by routine nursing measures is an aspect of normal care and basic patient maintenance, classical doctrines that were obscure and not fully understood are made clearer. It is now clearer to many in the Church that withholdings or removing these constitutes killing by omission. The Church is not getting onto a slippery slope by affirming this, but is making more articulate and clear an insight that has been vague and ambiguous for generations.

# CHAPTER SEVEN
# CATHOLIC ETHICS AND FEEDING THE COMATOSE

On March 15, 1986, the Judicial Council of the American Medical Association issued its opinion that the removal of food and water, provided by assisted means, from medically stable and nonterminal comatose patients should not be considered unethical or illegal.[1] In what could come to be a very influential article "The A.M.A. Statement on Tube Feeding: An Ethical Analysis", Fr. Kevin O'Rourke, O.P. argued in behalf of this opinion and has endorsed the legal and ethical permissibility of withdrawing nutrition and fluids from these patients.[2] His article is important, however, for the standards he proposes could very well become adopted by many Catholic health care institutions in the near future.

Fr. O'Rourke holds that the Judicial Council's Opinion is not objectionable, despite the fact that the Office of Pro-Life Activities of the National Conference of Catholic Bishops has endorsed other policies.[3] Fr. O'Rourke is probably the best exponent of the AMA's

---

[1] O'Rourke, O.P., Kevin. "The A.M.A. Statement on Tube Feeding: An Ethical Analysis", *America*, November 22, 1986. Pp. 321-323, 331. The title of his article is not fully accurate, for this statement emerged from the Judicial Council and there is no evidence that this opinion was endorsed by the membership at large of the American Medical Association.

[2] *Ibid.* P. 321.

[3] The Committee for Pro-Life Activities of the National Conference of Catholic bishops proposed the following "Guidelines for Legislation on Life-Sustaining Treatment":

> (g) Reaffirm public policies against homicide and assisted suicide. Medical treatment legislation may clarify procedures for discontinuing treatment which only secures a precarious and burdensome prolongation of life for the terminally ill patient, but should not condone or authorize any deliberate act or omission designed to cause a patient's death.
>
> (h) Recognize the presumption that certain basic measures such as nursing care, hydration, nourishment and the like must be maintained out of respect for the human dignity of every patient.
>
> (i) Protect the interests of innocent parties who are not competent to make treatment decisions on their own behalf. Life-sustaining treatment should not be discriminatorily withheld or withdrawn from mentally incompetent or retarded

new view as he is a highly regarded orthodox Catholic moralist and holds a great deal of influence over Catholic health institutions. Fr. O'Rourke supports the Judicial Council's opinion despite the fact that individual bishops in the nation have repeatedly spoken against it. Cardinal Joseph Bernardin and archbishop Phillip Hannan explicitly condemned the Judicial Council's opinion after it was issued.[4]

patients.

"Guidelines for Legislation on Life-Sustaining Treatment", National Conference of Catholic Bishops, November 10, 1984.

And in another statement issued by the NCCB, the following was stated:

Because human life has inherent value and dignity regardless of its condition, every patient should be provided with measures which can effectively preserve life without involving too grave a burden. Since food and water are necessities of life for all human beings, and can generally be provided without the risks and burdens of more aggressive means for sustaining life, the law should establish a strong presumption in favor of their use.

For most patients, measures for providing nourishment are morally obligatory even when other treatment can be withdrawn due to its burdensomeness or ineffectiveness.

Negative judgments about the "quality of life" of unconscious or otherwise disabled patients have led some in our society to propose withholding nourishment precisely in order to end these patients' lives. Society must take special care to protect against such discrimination. Laws dealing with medical treatment may have to take account of exceptional circumstances, when even means for providing nourishment may become too ineffective or burdensome to be obligatory. But such laws must establish clear safeguards against intentionally hastening the deaths of vulnerable patients by starvation or dehydration.

"Statement on Uniform Rights of the Terminally Ill Act", Committee for Pro-Life Activities, National Conference of Catholic Bishops, June 1986.

[4] Cardinal Bernardin wrote on April 18, 1986 in the *Chicago Catholic* that food and water were ordinary means that were to be given to the comatose and he said that the AMA Judicial Council's statement amounted to "legitimizing the denial of normal nourishment needed to sustain life." Archbishop Hannan's statement, issued on March 16, 1986, stated:

The Catholic Church has always held that families are not obligated to use extraordinary means -- such as artificial support systems -- to sustain the life

For example, Cardinal O'Connor called for the feeding of Nancy Ellen Jobes, Cardinal Law urged that Paul Brophy not be starved to death, and Archbishop Roger Mahony was highly critical of court decisions to allow Elizabeth Bouvia to be starved to death.[5] Fr. O'Rourke might think there is nothing objectionable about the new Judicial Council standard, but that opinion is being sharply questioned by many of our nation's bishops. And in October, the Catholic bishops of New Jersey issued the most forceful statement on this matter to date by filing a brief in the Nancy Ellen Jobes case which specifically opposes the removal of food and fluids from patients because of their apparent lack of mental ability.[6] In what follows I will summarize and criticize his fundamental arguments in support of the new Judicial Council's opinion, and then turn to his

of a patient in a hopelessly irreversible coma. However, food and water are ordinary means of sustaining life. Therefore, the Catholic Church opposes the American Medical Association position because it approves denying a person the normal nourishment that he or she needs to sustain life.

[5] On April 9, 1986, Cardinal O'Connor issued the following statement:

Regarding the Roman Catholic position on the requirements for medical treatments to prolong life, one must look to the report of the Pontifical Academy of Sciences, released October 30, 1985, which provides, in part, that in cases of permanent coma, irreversible as far as it is possible to predict, life prolonging medical intervention need not be employed, but care, including food and water, must be provided. If any prospect of recovery is medically established, treatment is required.

In the Paul Brophy case, Cardinal Law was quoted in the Boston *Globe* on June 9, 1985 in support of the New England Sinai Hospital which was arguing for his right to be fed. The Cardinal stated: "That position is consistent with what I believe are Catholic moral and medical practices."

Archbishop Roger Mahony criticized the California Second District Court of Appeal when it allowed a feeding tube to be removed from Elizabeth Bouvia. Archbishop Mahony stated that the Court had "entered a realm where its competence does not lie." He said that "If the reasoning of the court prevails, and a person is legally permitted to end his or her life because they perceive the quality of their life to be in adequate, are we far from the day when others -- doctors, family members, judges -- may actually 'order' the mercy killing of a person based on the same logic?"

[6] Brief, *amicus curiae*, New Jersey Catholic Conference, *In the Matter of Nancy Ellen Jobes*. This brief represents one Roman Catholic archdiocese, four Roman Catholic dioceses and one Byzantine Catholic diocese.

secondary assertions.

# A
# FUNDAMENTAL ARGUMENTS

## 1
## Criteria for Withdrawing Treatment

The most novel aspect of Fr. O'Rourke's defense of the Judicial Council's Opinion is his assertion that medical treatments can be removed "if the prolongation of life does not contribute to the attainment of the purpose of life."[7] He writes that "[T]here is no need to seek to remove the fatal pathology or to circumvent its effects if the efforts would not enable the individual to achieve cognitive-affective function and strive for the purpose of life".[8]

---

[7] O'Rourke, *art. cit.* P. 322. Joseph Fletcher makes much the point when he argues that there is no duty to provide medical treatment when the *humanum* point is crossed. This is the point at which the rational faculty is lost. See his: *To Live and to Die: When, Why and How.* (New York: Springer Verlag, 1973). Pp. 122 and 26-35.

[8] *Ibid.* While Fr. O'Rourke has made the best defense of the A.M.A's new opinion, the most effective argument made in behalf of removing food and water from medically stable patients is that traditional medical ethics has allowed this. Proponents of this viewpoint argue that the Roman Catholic medical ethical tradition has permitted food and water to be rejected by patients. Edward Bayer, for example has argued that Francisco De Vitoria (1486-1546) held that a sick person was obliged to take food if a hope of living a while was still present, but if the person was repulsed by food, then there was no obligation. He asserts that this viewpoint was also espoused by De Lugo and Ligouri. See: Bayer, Edward, "Is Food Always Obligatory?" in *Ethics and Medics*, Vol. 10, No. 9, September 1985, (Braintree, Mass: Pope John Center) P. 3. It seems, however, that the sorts of cases that Vitoria, De Lugo and Ligouri were citing were quite different from those now being debated. For in the Jobes, Brophy, Requena and Rasmussen cases, there was the prospect that these patients would live "a while" if not an indefinite period of time. Also, it could not be said that food was repulsive to these individuals. Beverly Requena declared that she did not wish to be fed, but she did not express a revulsion to food. She was repulsed by her paralyzed condition, and that is very different from being repulsed by food.

Even further, the social situation is very different now from that faced by the great fifteenth and sixteenth century moralists. It is not at all evident that they faced an international campaign to overturn laws against passive and active mercy killing. And if the dictum of the Second Vatican Council means anything that the Church read the signs of the times, it would seem to mean that this campaign be taken into consideration in the present context. It is becoming widely known that the euthanasia movement wishes

According to Fr. O'Rourke, to pursue this objective one must have the ability to function at the cognitive, affective and spiritual levels, and if efforts to restore functioning at this level are futile, there is no obligation to sustain physiological life.[9] Those without cognitive-affective function (and possibly "spiritual" function) who cannot strive for the purpose of life are still persons and human beings, but one wonders what practical weight is being given to this admonition.[10] Fr. O'Rourke claims that it is not any specific treatment, but the life of the person receiving the treatments, that becomes burdensome and which makes all life-sustaining treatments extraordinary. He suggests that physiological life is not sufficiently valuable in itself to warrant any measures whatsoever to continue its existence and he wants to adopt the theory that human life has its sanctity because of capabilities for rational functioning.[11] He asserts that in some senses it might be spiritually better for a person to die from cancer than to accept treatment.[12]

### Critique

Fr. O'Rourke does not apply these criteria consistently, for in some places he speaks only of a need for a cognitive and affective potential for functioning and elsewhere he speaks of a need for a

---

to gain legal and social endorsement for virtually forms of euthanasia by first gaining acceptance of living wills, and then of passive mercy killing by withdrawal of food and water, and finally euthanasia by lethal injections. To not take that "sign of the time" into consideration strikes this author as being pastorally irresponsible.

[9] *Ibid.*

[10] *Ibid.* P. 331. He states that those who suffer fatal pathologies are still persons who are not to be neglected.

[11] *Ibid.* P. 322. It should be noted that virtually the same claim was made by Fr. Richard McCormick, S.J., whom Fr. O'Rourke has criticized as being a modern voluntarist. It is difficult to see how Fr. O'Rourke can criticize Fr. McCormick for putting classical voluntarism in modern garb without also being criticized for doing the same.

[12] *Ibid.* P. 323.

spiritual potentiality for functioning.[13] His criteria for possessing the capability for striving for the purpose of life shift, as he holds at one point that all that is needed is a cognitive-affective capability, and in another place he implies that there must be some spiritual capability.[14] If there is a spiritual capability, whatever that might consist in, it would seem that those with chronic depression and suicidal tendencies cannot operate toward the purpose of life.

Fr. O'Rourke seems to believe that the comatose are so clearly different from other categories of patients that criteria can be used to permit withdrawing all treatment from them would also justify withdrawing treatment from these other classes as well. He fails to see that it is very difficult to make accurate diagnoses of many patients who are neurologically unresponsive. He claims that those in deep coma do not experience pain, but he dismiss the fact that the neurological diagnosis of "deep coma" is very ambiguous and difficult to make. By failing to see this, he is putting many severely brain-damaged persons in danger of an excruciating death by starvation or dehydration.

His criteria in fact demand that an arbitrarily defined level of neurological functioning be established before imposing any duties to give assisted food and water to the medically vulnerable. Doing this is contrary to recent developments in law, and it would be contrary to the principles of the Older Americans Act.[15] It would seem that many mentally impaired patients would fit into the category of patients for whom cognitive-affective function cannot be restored and who "cannot strive for the purpose of life."

One must ask why those with diminished physical capacity to strive for human goals should be included in the category of

---

[13] For example, in one place he says that "[P]hysiological function bereft of the potential for cognitive-affective function does not benefit the patient and does not contribute to pursuing the purpose of life". Elsewhere he says that pursuing the goals of life requires not only cognitive and affective function but also functioning at the spiritual level. Is there a difference? *Ibid.* P. 322.

[14] *Ibid.* P. 322.

[15] *The Older Americans Act of 1965*, 42 U.S.C. 3001 (1982). Among other things, this act holds that older Americans are to be provided with whatever medical care and treatment is necessary to enable them to function at their highest mental and physical levels possible.

patients from which virtually all forms of care and treatment can permissibly be removed?[16] Fr. O'Rourke wishes to limit his standard to those who lack cognitive or affective potential, but people such as cerebral palsy victim Elizabeth Bouvia who argues that their bodies are useless, implying that they cannot strive for human goals in their useless bodies. Why could not she ask for removal of all treatments by invoking O'Rourke's criteria? Many disabled would ask why only mental disability should count.

Fr. O'Rourke fails to see that his ambiguous criteria pose a very serious threat to the handicapped and mentally ill in our state institutions, who are among the least protected members of our society. Do the severely demented, severely retarded or seriously schizophrenic people also lack the "spiritual" capability to strive for the human goals? Do chronically depressed persons who desire suicide also lack the spiritual or affective potential to pursue the goals of life? Should those with advanced Alzheimer's disease, advanced senile dementia, advanced multiple sclerosis, advanced Huntington's Chorea and advanced Parkinson's dementia of Guam also be placed in this category because they have supposedly lost this capacity? Fr. O'Rourke seems to think that affective or spiritual potential for human striving is a clear-cut category, but that is simply not so. Their capacity to "strive for the purposes of life" is certainly limited, and one wonders why they cannot have their nutrition and fluids withdrawn. Why should not suicidal individuals who lack the affective capability to pursue human goals have a "right" to have food and water removed that is equal to that of the comatose?

Fr. O'Rourke considers judgments about the burdens of life to be complex and difficult, but he does not let this deter him from urging that such judgments be made. Having acknowledge this, he does not affirm the need to take a more protective course of action.

---

[16] This is a reasonable question because persons do not strive for human goals simply by cognitive or affective means, but also by bodily means. Fr. O'Rourke implicitly holds that the only important human goals are those which are not achieved through bodily actions, and he demeans the importance of the body in human life. He implies that physiological life is of insignificant value, but a more balanced approach must hold that there is some form of mysterious human life and vitality present in the persistently unconscious person--a life that we do not fully understand--but which must not be deliberately destroyed by either omission or commission.

From the viewpoint of the law, these judgments are not merely difficult, but impossible, and anyattempt to make them becomes discriminatory and unjust. If the "fundamental option for the poor" means anything, it would mean that criteria for medical decision making would favor provision of care and prohibit judgments about the "burden of their lives."

According to Fr. O'Rourke, there is no duty to sustain "mere physiological life". One must question this claim because it degrades the value of physiological life. He holds that it has so little independent value to "mere physiological life" that there is no moral duty to sustain it when other (psychological?) capabilities have been suppressed. And it seems that this view is contrary to the classical Catholic view which held that membership in the human species gives human life its sanctity.[17]

Fr. O'Rourke says that treatment could be withdrawn if the life of the individual receiving it was very burdensome because the withdrawal of feeding would only increase the burdens of the person's life. But this lacks clarity because withdrawing feeding would only increase burdens involved in the life of the person. His view is even more rationally indefensible if one presumes that the comatose cannot experience their environment. And if the person is able to experience his or her environment, it would seem that providing food and water would be mandatory because of the agony that is associated with their withdrawal.

It is claimed by Fr. O'Rourke that it might be spiritually better for a cancer patient to reject treatment than to continue

---

[17] Dr. William May has argued well that it is membership in the human species that establishes the "worth" of the human being. Speaking of feral children, he commented:

> When these human offspring - beings *certainly* human by reason of their membership in the human species and, in my judgment (and, I believe, in Christian faith) infinitely precious beings imaging the living God - were found by other human beings and brought back in to human community, it was evident that they had no realization or awareness of themselves as selves.

The point he is making is that the value of the person is based on being born into the human species, and not in possessing the ability to make our powers of reason functional or operative, as O'Rourke would hold. See: William E. May, *Human Existence, Medicine and Ethics*, P. 30.

living, but would it be better for a cancer victim to reject food and water in order to precipitate death than to continue living? This question, which Fr. O'Rourke fails to answer, is important because it is conceivable that such cancer patients might be closer to death than are some comatose patients. Fr. O'Rourke hints that it would be "spiritually" better to starve a comatose patient, but how could it be "spiritually" better to starve someone to death who cannot strive after life's goals? How can it be "better" to certainly end the life of an innocent person by denying food and water than to continue their life by providing minimal care? If such a person is incapable of "spiritual" striving, it would seem that giving them readily providable, successful, nonpainful assisted feeding would do them no "spiritual" harm either.

Fr. O'Rourke asserts that the "end" of life cannot be attained without potential for spiritual and cognitive and affective function. This claim demands that two questions be answered. First, in a Christian framework, should not the issue be whether the individual stands in a relation to God rather than to human goals? And second, can we thus be sure that the comatose are not striving for salvation even in their severely damaged condition? The fundamental problem with this criterion is that it leaves the critical term "purpose of life" materially undefined and he does not establish an index specifying when a person actually has the power to strive for these goals. There are simply no objective criteria to determine when this capability exists, and certainly no criteria that would be admissible in a court of law, as O'Rourke optimistically thinks there would be.

Despite this, Fr. O'Rourke apparently wants physicians to use this criterion so that some classes of patients can be eased out of this life, but he does not see that this criterion will permit other classes of patients to also be eased out by the omission of food and water. This failure creates the specter of physicians debating among themselves the nature, meaning and purpose of life before providing care and treatment. Fr. O'Rourke is experienced enough to know that most, if not all, physicians do not want this and are incapable of resolving in this sort of debate.

## 2
### The Nature of Assisted Feeding

Fr. O'Rourke asserts that "[W]ithholding artificial hydration and nutrition from a patient in an irreversible coma does not introduce a new fatal pathology; rather it allows an already existing fatal pathology to take its natural course".[18] He holds that comatose patients who die after food and water are withdrawn do so because of their inability to swallow.[19] He asserts that decisions to provide assisted feeding should be decided on the basis of the presence of a fatal pathology: ". . . when making ethical or legal decisions concerning the care of persons in an irreversible coma or with other serious pathological conditions, rather than discussing whether death is imminent or whether the patient is terminally ill, we should ask whether a fatal pathology is present."[20] He suggests that the important issue in determining whether assisted feeding should be given to medically stable but comatose patients is not how long the patient will live with feeding, but whether there is an obligation to provide life-support systems to the seriously ill.[21] He claims that "[L]ife prolonging therapy aims at removing a potentially fatal pathology--for example, surgery for cancer--or aims at circumventing

---

[18] *Ibid.* P. 322.

[19] *Ibid.*

[20] *Ibid.* While he is not clear on this issue, he holds that life-sustaining therapies remove, circumvent or delay a fatal pathology. He holds that with the comatose there is no obligation to give any life-sustaining therapy or care whatsoever with the exception of hygienic care. But if assisted feeding can *delay* death by starvation and dehydration, why should it not be mandatory, just as we would presume insulin injections for a permanently comatose patient would be obligatory. O'Rourke has not suggested that comatose diabetics be killed by withdrawal of insulin, and it is not clear why assisted feeding should be viewed differently from insulin therapy.

[21] *Ibid.* P. 321. "The important issue is not how long the patient might live with life support systems, but whether the life support system should be applied to seriously ill patients in the first place." This is not quite true. If some life support systems are withdrawn from certain classes of "seriously ill patients" (whomever they might be) that withdrawal might be morally equivalent to killing by omission precisely because the patients could live a good length of time with that system. For example, many young people who are seriously ill with respiratory ailments can live many productive years with newly developed "backpack" respirators that are relatively nonburdensome, risk-free and inexpensive to maintain. Precisely because they can live many years with those devices, to refuse to provide them would be to kill these students by omission. O'Rourke has failed to make this important and necessary distinction in his desire to defend the new A.M.A. decision.

or delaying the effects of the fatal pathology.[22]

[22] *Ibid*. P. 322. Fr. O'Rourke has so expanded the category of medical treatments that the has all but virtually eliminated the traditional category of "normal care." This category has included those elements of patient maintenance which enabled a patient to cope more fully with his conditions and included hygienic care, protection from exposure, provision of food and water and psychological support. If food and water are medical treatments that remove potentially fatal pathologies, then why do we not define hunger and thirst as fatal pathologies and therefore clinical conditions, we should prepare ourselves for a radical change in traditional medical practice. Hunger and thirst are not clinical conditions, even though in their extreme states they can precipitate clinical conditions. The need for food and water is a basic need of the body, just as are the needs for sanitary care and protection from exposure. Meeting these needs is not a medical treatment, but is an aspect of basic patient maintenance. Assisted feeding no more inhibits or remedies potentially fatal pathologies than does a urinary catheter, and neither are medical treatments so much as they are elements of patient maintenance or basic nursing care.

In his testimony before the New Jersey Bioethics Commission on August 19, 1987, Dr. Stephen Miles, M.D., the Associate Director of the Center for Clinical Ethics at the University of Chicago, said the following:

> The equation of nourishment with treatment--was *constructed* in order to allow for the discontinuation of nourishment--by analogy to now widely accepted arguments for the use of other life-sustaining medical treatments, like respirators. This equation works this way. First, it makes the act of feeding--as morally inert as a respirator. Second, it focuses the evaluation of nourishment on the disabled person and their disease and makes other considerations--including the moral perceptions of family or health care providers of secondary importance.
>
> The equation of nourishment with treatment is proposed as a premise for the family to learn, not as a conclusion that [sic] family arrives at. With the equation of feeding with medical treatment, a certain moral perception and family authority is imposed on patients and families as the symbolic moral understandings of families are voided as medically uninformed, as emotive, rather than emotive claims.
>
> Families who reject the feeding-treatment equation and claim that feeding is a fundamental interpersonal caring transaction are adopting what has been termed the symbolic argument. The symbolic claim and families who hold to it have been dismissed in mainstream literature on this subject. Such families are seen as denying illness, afraid of death, engaging in primitive thinking (by one prominent ethicist, who should have known better, as violating the autonomy of their loved one.)

Fr. O'Rourke contends that nasogastric feeding can become burdensome to a comatose patient just as medical treatments can become burdensome to a cancer patient.[23] There is an obligation to provide comfort and spiritual care for those patients from whom assisted feeding is withdrawn.[24]

### Critique

There is an important difference between a public policy that equates nourishment with other medical treatments thereby permitting the discontinuation of nourishment and one that simply entrusts the care of the comatose or profoundly demented persons to loving, involved family members, who are to decide within the family--the terms of their decisions. To understand what is at stake, I will outline the difference between nourishment and medical treatments.

Treatments are medical interventions, designed to affect health. Treatments are outside of our customary experience. They are based on an arcane and specialized knowledge. They are given by special authorities in special settings. These authorities exercise considerable influence over the judgment to use treatment in that they are accorded special wisdom to determine whether a given therapy is medically futile, indicated, or contraindicated. Individual treatments are familiar to only a small percentage of persons. Morally, the individual is responsible for his own health, and is the principle authority as to whether treatments are used. I call this medical treatment of nourishment, "alimentation".

The ethics of feeding differs from the ethics of medical treatment. Within family transactions, we share ourselves in a collective identity, we participate in creating and maintaining shared symbolic understandings of our actions and interactions. Though from outside the family, our actions appear to express an unrestricted autonomy, from within a family we know better, we are willingly connected and bound by the integrity of the family duties and the family vision, a deep respect for the family way.

---

[23] *Ibid.* P. 322. Fr. O'Rourke holds that treatments, including assisted feeding, can become burdensome insofar as the pursuing of the purpose of life is concerned. But should it not be asked if the withdrawal of food and water can also become burdensome, and if so, should not those burdens be weighed against the burdens of a life that cannot pursue the goal of life?

[24] *Ibid.* P. 322. "There is an ethical obligation to keep the person comfortable . . ." "Maintaining that the life of a person need not be prolonged when a fatal pathology is present does not mean that the person should be neglected." P. 331.

It is Fr. O'Rourke's opinion that the need for assisted feeding is a fatal condition, but if this need is a fatal condition, should he not also other conditions such as a diabetics' need for insulin also be seen as a as a fatal condition? Should not the need for sanitary care or protection from exposure also be considered as a fatal condition as is the need for feeding?

By holding this, he has established a standard which will allow many more kinds of patients than just the comatose to have life-sustaining food and water withdrawn. Many seriously handicapped, debilitated, senile and demented patients are unable to take food and fluids orally. Should we consider all of these patients as suffering from a fatal pathology as well? His definition of life-prolonging therapies as those which prevent inhibit life-threatening conditions is probably an accurate description of the function of medical therapies and procedures, but it fails to see that there are some procedures that must be offered by health care providers to all patients, irrespective of their clinical conditions. Implied in his view of the nature of assisted feeding is the understanding that assisted feeding is a medical treatment and is not an aspect of normal care. Assisted feeding is not a medical treatment but is an aspect of normal care because its immediate, proximate and direct finality is not to cure, remedy or palliate *clinical conditions*, but to meet the natural need of the body for extrinsic natural bodily resources.[25] Indirectly and remotely, food and water might serve other purposes, but their primary end is to meet the needs of the body--any body, sick or healthy--for food and water.[26]

These aspects of basic patient maintenance have traditionally consisted of: 1) protection from exposure; 2) hygienic care or sanitary care; and, 3) provision of nutrition and fluids. These procedures merely sustain the normal bodily functions of the patient

---

[25] See: Barry, O.P., Robert, "Facing Hard Cases: The Ethics of Assisted Feeding" *Issues in Law and Medicine*, Vol. 2, No. 2. Pp. 100-106.

[26] See: Barry, "The Ethics of Providing Life Sustaining Nutrition and Fluids to Incompetent Patients", *The Journal of Family and Culture*, Vol. 1, No. 2. P. 27.

and support the natural bodily defenses of the person.[27] These are different from medical treatments because they do not directly and immediately impede the course of already-existing pathological conditions.[28] Traditionally, they have been provided to all patients whenever there was a need for them, which is indicated by the fact that consent is not ordinarily required to provide them.[29] And any facility which deliberately decided to withhold these from patients would be guilty of serious neglect and abuse.

The Vatican's "Declaration on Euthanasia" stated that euthanasia was "an act or an omission which of itself or by intention causes death, in order that suffering may in this way be eliminated".[30] The critical issue in decisions to provide assisted feeding to the medically stable comatose is that when the provision of food and water through routine and customary nursing procedures can meet the needs of the body in a meaningful way the failure to provide them is morally equivalent to killing by omission.[31] But if the withdrawal of feeding provided by these measures will not have any impact on the clinical picture of the patient, or if the provision of assisted feeding by nursing procedures would only sustain life for a minimal period of time (a few hours or days), then its provision

---

[27] See: Piccione, Joseph, "The Tradition of Care", *The Euthanasia Review*, Vol. 1, No. 2. Pp. 129-131.

[28] Barry, O.P., "The Ethics of Providing Life-Sustaining Nutrition and Fluids to Incompetent Patients". P. 27.

[29] Piccione, *Op. cit.* P. 130. He notes that feeding traditionally has not been provided if the patient was imminently dying, if the feeding was futile or if the feeding process itself caused grave burdens. In all other circumstances, however, the tradition of care required the provision of food and water to patients.

[30] Sacred Congregation for the Doctrine of the Faith, "Declaration on Euthanasia". (Washington, D.C: United States Catholic Conference, 1980.)

[31] O'Rourke rejects this and holds that determining the obligation to give treatment is the central issue, but this is too ambiguous. To determine the obligation, one must know precisely the condition of the patient, the life expectancy of the patient and the nature of the treatments being offered.

is not such a kind of culpable killing.[32]

  Fr. O'Rourke's claim that the comatose condition resulting in difficulties in swallowing causes the death of the individual after food and water have been removed is like saying that a diabetic dies from diabetes after successfully administered insulin is withdrawn from the diabetic. This is false, for if a diabetic dies after removal of insulin, it is the choice to no longer provide it that is the cause of death and not the diabetes. Similarly, when a comatose but medically stable person dies consequent to the removal of assisted feeding given through ordinary nursing care techniques, it is the effect of that choice, and not the comatose condition or the inability to swallow that causes death. People die from coma when their neurological condition deteriorates so badly that their major organ systems fail. But when persons dies after nutrition and fluids are withdrawn, they die as a result of dehydration or starvation, and coma is not the fundamental and proximate cause of death.

  One must ask Fr. O'Rourke how it is that coma actually kills, given the fact that the symptoms associated with death from starvation appear to be identical to the kind of death he attributes to coma. It is very easy to see how definitive denial of food and water kill a medically stable individual, but it is not clear how a coma kills one. When their food and water are withdrawn, these patients die from a positive decision to do nothing whatsoever to help them survive.

  Coma by itself is not any more of a lethal pathology than is diabetes when minimal attention is given to it. Coma and other clinical conditions of these patients only become fatal when a decision is made to abandon all care and treatment of them, and they would not die except for such a decision. Were these patients to be provided food and water as are all other medically stable patients, their lives would not be in jeopardy. And one must ask him what the proximate cause of death is of patients who have

---

[32] Dennis Horan discusses the legal and ethical implications of withdrawing feeding in his article "Failure to Feed: An Ethical and legal Discussion", *Issues in Law and Medicine*, Vol. 2, No. 2. He argues that the legal doctrine of proximate causation should be accepted in both the legal and ethical debates. This doctrine "creates responsibility for injury for any action or omission when *but for* the happening of that action or omission, the injury would not have resulted. In addition, the act must not be excessively remote from the injury sustained". P. 150.

feeding tubes removed. He has not taken into consideration the doctrine of the "Declaration on Euthanasia" which holds that an act or omission causing death by itself or intentionally to eliminate suffering constitutes euthanasia.

## B
## SECONDARY CLAIMS

### 1
### Personhood and the Duty to Feed

Fr. O'Rourke argues that those who lack a cognitive, affective and spiritual potential to strive for human purposes are still persons, but it is hard to see how this can be the case.[33] If individuals who have no cognitive and affective capacity and cannot strive for spiritual values are now merely a mass of "physiological functions", what does it entail in O'Rourke's approach to say that they are still persons? Fr. O'Rourke implies that they cannot act toward human finalities, they lack the highest and most distinguishing traits of persons, and their physical lives are of such little value that they cannot warrant any care or treatment. It seems difficult to see why one should continue to call them human persons in a meaningful sense. As we shall see later, Dr. D. Alan Shewmon, M.D. is more forthright and has argued that such individuals are "humanoid animals" and claimed that it was permissible even to put them painlessly to death as one does with animals.[34] Fr. O'Rourke would be more consistent if he concurred with Shewmon's analysis and held that they were humanoid animals toward whom there are no duties whatsoever.

### 2
### Revising the Roman Catholic Medical-Ethical Criteria

Fr. O'Rourke holds that ". . .[T]he degree of pain is not per

---

[33] O'Rourke, *art. cit.* P. 331.

[34] Shewmon, M.D., D. Alan. "The Metaphysics of Brain Death, Persistent Vegetative State and Dementia", *The Thomist*, Vol. 49, No. 1. Pp. 29-81.

se a consideration in the ethical decision concerning useless therapy; neither should it influence the legal decision concerning the same issue. The degree of pain may influence the decision concerning the burden that prolonging life may entail, but not concerning the usefulness or uselessness of life-prolonging therapy."[35] It is unclear why he would give consideration to pain as a factor in judging whether a feeding tube should be provided, for he rejects pain as a criterion for its provision. It seems that he wants to eliminate the question of the pain involved in feeding totally. Fr. O'Rourke realizes that invoking the issue of pain makes the case for feeding the comatose even stronger. For, if comatose patients cannot experience pain, then feeding them is no burden at least in that regard. But if they can experience pain, then denying food and water will impose severe pain on them.

Fr. O'Rourke's rejection of the traditional criterion of physical pain in favor of the "burden of life" standard is a frank endorsement of quality-of-life judgments.[36] Traditional Roman Catholic medical ethics held that care or treatment became extraordinary if they caused severe pain, were difficult to provide or receive, were questionable in terms of benefits or were so costly that

---

[35] O'Rourke, *art. cit.* P. 323.

[36] Richard McCormick articulated the classical "quality-of-life" argument in Roman Catholic medical ethics in his article "To Save or Let Die: The Dilemma of Modern Medicine" where he said that:

> ". . .it is the kind of, quality of life thus saved (painful, poverty-stricken and deprived, away from home and friends, oppressive) that establishes a means as extraordinary. *That* type of life would be an excessive hardship for the individual. It would distort and jeopardize his grasp of the over-all meaning of life. Why? Because, it can be argued, human relationships--which are the very possibility of growth in love of God and neighbor--would be so threatened, strained, or submerged that they would no longer function as the heart and meaning of the individual's life as they should.

Fr. McCormick also argues that the potentiality of handicapped infants for meaningful human relationships should be a factor in deciding whether to provide medical treatments. It is very difficult to see how O'Rourke's criteria differ in any meaningful way from this classical "quality-of-life" standard. See: McCormick, S.J., Richard. "To Save or Let Die" in *How Brave a New World?*, (New York: Doubleday, 1981) P. 347-49.

a family could not meet its ordinary family obligations.[37] According to Fr. O'Rourke, pain is not an operative factor in determining whether treatments should be given to patients "without a potential for cognitive-affective function and the power to strive for the purpose of life". In claiming this, he is radically revising the traditional Catholic medical-ethical principles.

Fr. O'Rourke argues that those who cannot strive for human goals have lives that are burdensome and it is warranted to remove all care and treatment. What if that burden is not experienced by the person, as we presume with the comatose? How can we justly remove care if there is no experience of this burden? It seems to me that Fr. O'Rourke has to demonstrate that the lives of the comatose are burdensome to themselves and that the sufferings they experience warrant withholding the minimal care necessary to provide nasogastric feeding, which he has not done.

Paradoxically, Fr. O'Rourke denies that there is any obligation to provide food and water to a medically stable comatose person, but he holds that there is an obligation to provide comfort care that is evidently and patently futile. It is senseless to give "comfort care" to individuals who Fr. O'Rourke presumes to be beyond any experience of comfort or pain and who are being brought to death by denial of a crucial aspect of care. If a person is starving or dehydrating to death, giving them hygienic care and protection from exposure is certainly futile, and yet O'Rourke holds that it is obligatory to give such care. It would seem that such "cosmetic care" would be more for the benefit of the staff and family than for the patient, as it could persuade them that they are actually providing humane care for the patient. He paradoxically demands that comfort care be given, even though he admits that the evidence that the comatose feel pain is doubtful. If they have no ability to feel pain, then comfort care would obviously be futile! If there is no duty to provide assisted feeding, why is there a duty to provide these other forms of care? One suspects that he wants comfort care to be given to salve the consciences of those who decide to hurry the "biologically tenacious" along their way.

---

[37] Pope Pius XII, "Prolongation of Life: Allocution to an International Congress of Anesthesiologists", November 24, 1957, *The Pope Speaks*, Vol. 4. Pp. 393-398.

## 3
## Decision-Making for the Incompetent

Fr. O'Rourke suggests that denial of provision of food and water by proxies for handicapped infants if the children show no capacity to strive after human goals is morally legitimate.[38] He states this obliquely, but he explicitly holds that there is no obligation to provide medical treatment, (presumably including food and water) when these children have a fatal pathology because the burden of prolonged life of these children makes even food and water extraordinary.[39] And he holds that prolonging the life of an infant with a fatal disease might be unethical because it might cause grave burdens to the infant while striving for the purpose of life. While Fr. O'Rourke does not explicitly state that handicapped children should not be fed, it is hard not to infer this judgment from the context of this article. But like his other principles, this too is unacceptable, for if handicapped infants cannot strive for human goals, they do not know it, and by simply being alive, it can be claimed that they are striving for human goals. Their supposed incapacity is not a burden to them, and bringing them to death by dehydration or starvation creates rather than alleviates burdens for them. His view is unacceptable because it ignores the clear mandate to feed the hungry without any qualification or condition. In paragraph 69 of *Gaudium et Spes* the Council Fathers held that if a person is dying from hunger and one does not feed the person, those who have failed to feed him have killed him: "Feed the man dying of hunger, because if you do not feed him, you are killing him".[40]

Fr O'Rourke implies in his discussion of the care and treatment of handicapped infants that proxies should be free to

---

[38] O'Rourke, *art. cit.* Pp. 323, 331.

[39] *Ibid.*

[40] See: *The Documents of Vatican II*, edited by Austin Flannery, O.P., "Gaudium et Spes", para. 69. It should be noted that this statement was found first in the writings of the great canonist Gratian, and it is surprising that Fr. O'Rourke, a noted American canonist, has not taken account of this. See: Gratian, *Decretum*, c. 21, dist. LXXXVI: ed. Freiberg I, 302.

order withdrawal of food and water from any patient judged to be incapable of striving for human goals because of a lack of the cognitive, affective and spiritual capability to do so. This is too elastic a criterion to be ethically acceptable as it would put a large number of medically vulnerable individuals at risk.

While Fr. O'Rourke believes that proxy decisions for comatose patients should be made according to the criteria he establishes, he gives no indications as to how these criteria are to be instituted into law. He does not tell us how the law is to determine if a person who has died as a result of the withdrawal of food and water had the ability to strive for the purpose of life. O'Rourke has not been able to provide adequate ethical norms that can be translated into workable legal norms.

## Conclusion

We should recall that in this discussion that thousands and thousands of people every year receive assisted feeding. The American Society for Parenteral and Enteral Nutrition reported that more than 500,000 people received parenteral nutrition in the United States in 1984 and more than 780,000 received enteral nutrition that year.[41] And nearly half of those receiving enteral nutrition during that year were over 65.[42] Half of the patients receiving nutritional support, or almost two thirds of a million people suffered some sort of central nervous system damage such as stroke, and thus they might very well fit into Fr. O'Rourke's category of those lacking the cognitive-affective potential to strive for the purpose of human life.

Fr. O'Rourke's endorsement of the Judicial Council's opinion should is an unjustified intrusion of quality of life and proportionalist moral analysis into Catholic medical thought, and it should not be welcomed because of its failure to give due consideration to its consequences for the disabled, despairing and medically vulnerable. It should also be rejected because of its failure

---

[41] *Update*, American Society for Parenteral and Enteral Nutrition, Vol. 8, No. 4. P. 8.

[42] *Ibid*.

to answer a number of crucial questions and because of the risk it poses to many thousands of medically vulnerable persons in our society.

# CHAPTER EIGHT
# BRAIN DEATH, ENSOULMENT AND CARE

Dr. D. Alan Shewmon, M.D. argued recently that those who have lost cortical function, the brain dead, permanently unconscious, comatose those suffering dementia, and hydroencephalic infants lack a rational soul as this is understood in Thomistic natural philosophy.[1] Because these individuals have lost cortical function, they have lost the capability for rational thought, do not have a rational soul and should not be considered as human persons, but as "humanoid animals".[2]

Because they do not have the capability for rational thought, their bodies are incompatible with the human essence.[3] He compares these individuals to "brainless vegetative substances".[4] Failing to meet the criteria for the possession of a rational soul, he argues that if there were sufficient reasons it would be permissible to withdraw all medical treatments, nutrition and fluids from these individuals, and give them lethal injections to "painlessly" put them to sleep as if they were animals if there were sufficient reasons.[5] Even further, he argues that bringing these individuals to death would be mandatory in some instances.[6] Dr. Shewmon argues that those who have lost all brain function, are clearly and certainly dead and that this opinion is now universally accepted in the medical community.

---

[1] Shewmon, M.D., D., Alan. "The Metaphysics of Brain Death, Persistent Vegetative State and Dementia". *The Thomist*, Vol. 49, No. 1, Pp. 24-81.

[2] *Ibid*. P. 59. Shewmon ascribes this only to the demented, but in so doing, he implicitly attributes it to the comatose, persistently unconscious, brain dead and hydroencephalic.

[3] *Ibid*. P. 60.

[4] *Ibid*. P. 46.

[5] *Ibid*. P. 73.

[6] *Ibid*. P. 79. The purpose would be to allow the cadaver "to be piously buried" so that the family could "end their anxiety and uncertainty, begin their mourning process, and go on with their lives again." Despite assertions that word games not be played with cadavers, Shewmon strangely calls for the removal of life support from cadavers.

This claim should not be accepted at face value, for leading medical practitioners, ethicists and philosophers are now seriously questioning whether those who are "brain dead" are fully dead.

The leading proponents of this critical view have been Dr. Paul Byrne, Peter Salsich, Fr. Paul Quay, and the late Dr. Sean O'Reilly.[7] They have argued that the brain dead are not yet fully dead but are only in the last stages of dying and should be treated as living human beings. To understand this perspective, the following case should be noted.

The Journal of the American Medical Association reported the case of a young woman who was involved in an automobile accident and was brought to the emergency room with severe head injuries.[8] The woman was pregnant with a 24 week-old baby, and it was hoped that her life could be sustained long enough long enough to save the child's life. Four days after admission, she was diagnosed as being certainly brain dead according to the strictest standards of brain death. Nonetheless, she was given intravenous feeding and antibiotics, and a week later, her baby was delivered by Caesarean section. It is very difficult to believe that a "dead" person could gestate a child for as long as she did. Physician Mark Siegler and ethicist Daniel Wikler commented that it is because of these sorts of cases that some physicians are having serious doubts as to whether those who loose whole brain function are necessarily dead:

> It has been known for some time that brain-dead patients, suitably maintained, can breathe, circulate blood, digest food, evacuate wastes, maintain body temperature, generate new tissue and fulfill other functions as well. All of this is remarkable in a "corpse". Granted, these functions could not be maintained without artificial aid and, even so, will cease within a few weeks. However, many living patients depend on machines and will not live long;

---

[7] These views have been promoted most fully in an article "Brain Death - The Patient, The Physician and Society", *Gonzaga Law Review*, Vol. 18, 1982-3, #13, pp. 429-516.

[8] Dillon, *et. al.* "Life Support and Maternal Brain Death During Pregnancy", *Journal of the American Medical Association*, Vol. 248, No. 9, pp. 1088-1095.

they are not thereby classified as (already) dead.

Now we are told that the brain-dead patient can nurture a child in the womb, which permits live birth several weeks "postmortem". Perhaps this is the straw that breaks the conceptual camel's back. It becomes irresistible to speak of brain-dead patients being "somatically alive" (what sort of "nonsomatic death" is the implied alternative?), of being "terminally ill", and eventually of "dying". These are different ways of saying that such patients (or at least, their bodies) are alive. The death of the brain seems not to serve as the boundary; it is a tragic, ultimately fatal loss, but not death itself. Bodily death occurs, later, when integrated functioning ceases.[9]

Shewmon's claims need to be challenged, for he is probably the most articulate exponent of the theory that the brain dead are truly dead and that there are no responsibilities to continue providing care and treatment for them. In this section, I shall argue that it is merely a conjectural opinion that the individuals in the conditions he describes do not have rational souls, that even in their deeply debilitated states they still have moral rights not to be directly killed and that it not even tolerable, much less mandatory, to take directly lethal acts or omissions against them. It will be argued that it is not always and everywhere immoral to remove life-sustaining medical treatments from these patients, but that it is required that they be given life-sustaining food and fluids when this is medically possible and that they be free from any deliberately and directly lethal actions.

To do this, I will first review some medical issues and developments that Dr. Shewmon has refrained from mentioning. While Shewmon has shown a great deal of familiarity with recent developments in medicine and the treatment of hydroencephalic infants, the comatose, persistently unconscious, and brain dead, he

---

[9] Siegler, Mark., and Daniel Wikler, "Brain Death and Life Birth", *Journal of the American Medical Association*, Sept. 3, 1982, Vol. 248, No. 9. Pp. 1101-2.

appears to be unfamiliar with some other developments that are pertinent to his theories. These have a direct bearing on his claims that these individuals are "humanoid animals" and on the ethical judgments he makes about their treatment. Then I will discuss his views about the nature of the rational soul to show that they are not fully expressive of the principles of Thomistic natural philosophy. Finally, I will analyze his assertions concerning the manner in which these various classes of patients are to be treated.

Dr. Shewmon's article has raised a number of medical and ethical issues about the status of the brain dead, their diagnosis and their treatment. In what follows, I wish to give consideration to some of these problems.

In 1968, the *Harvard Committee on Brain Death* established criteria for diagnosing brain death by requiring that such a diagnosis only be made if two physicians confirm that the patient had a flat EEG, was unresponsive to external stimuli, showed no signs of spontaneous respiration or muscular movement, showed no brain or spinal reflexes, was not hypothermic or under CNS depressants, and had been diagnosed as being in this condition for twenty four hours.[10] The medical, legal and social endorsement of brain death criteria have enabled physicians to transplant organs and have permitted families to be spared the emotional exhaustion and financial burden of coping with patients who were sustained with minimal care. But serious questions remain concerning the reliability of criteria for diagnosing brain death and about the treatment of the brain dead. May one remove assisted feeding from the brain dead? May their organs be removed and transplanted to others? May they be given lethal injections to bring them to "somatic death"?

Brain death criteria have had the effect of creating a whole new class of patients who are somewhat dead but do not act like other dead individuals. While the brain dead are purportedly dead, many are reluctant to treat them as others who are dead are treated because often they breathe and respirate independently like other

---

[10] Beecher, Henry, K. "A Definition of Irreversible Coma. Report of the Ad Hoc Committee of the Harvard Medical School to Examine the Definition of Brain Death." *Journal of the American Medical Association*, No. 205, (1968) Pp. 337-40.

living human beings.[11] Some have suggested that the brain dead were not truly dead, but experience what they call "somatic death", the death of the vegetative functions of the body, had yet to occur.[12] Somatic death is not true death, but is simply the final stage of the death that began with the demise of the brain.

As a result of the development of these and other brain death criteria, the problem of how to understand, care for and treat the brain dead or "neomorts" has arisen. Neomorts are individuals who are supposedly brain dead, and yet many show some remarkable signs of vitality. Commenting on the treatment of neomorts, Debbie Salamone noted that:

> Scientists say neomorts give doctors a chance to test new drugs and medical procedures before they use them on living patients.
>
> Neomorts are a source of transplantable organs and provide storage place [sic] for organs until a recipient can be found. They also help surgeons learn new medical techniques as well as substitute for some of the more than 90 million animals used for scientific research each year.
>
> [I]n 1981, surgeons at Temple University in Philadelphia put the Jarvik-7 artificial heart into the *functioning bodies* (italics mine) of five brain-dead people to test ways to

---

[11] Douglas Walton refrains from admitting that they should be buried as others who are considered dead, and he takes great pains to argue that they should be treated differently from others who are dead. See his: *Brain Death: Ethical Considerations*. (West Lafayette, Indiana: Purdue Indiana Press, 1980) pp. 2-4. Currie also reported that Elizabeth Kubler Ross claimed that some patients with flat EEG's actually heard their death notices being pronounced. See: Currie, Bethia, S. "The Redefinition of Death" in *Organism, Medicine and Metaphysics*. Edited by Spicker, Stuart, F. (Dordrecht: Reidel, 1978) Walton claims that angiography can be used to supplement EEGs, but he admits that these procedures are highly invasive and when used occasionally they do not facilitate diagnosis. Richard Doerflinger noted that the brain dead have been known to develop pneumonia and even bed sores as well. See: Doerflinger, Richard. "Resource Paper: Definition of Death Legislation", National Conference of Catholic Bishops, Committee on Pro-Life Activities, 1983, p. 28.

[12] Siegler, Mark,. and Wikler, Daniel. "Brain Death and Live Birth", p. 1101.

implant the device.

Dr. Jack Kolff, chief of cardiothoracic surgery at Temple and principle investigator during the neomort surgery, said doctors probably would not have been able to successfully implant the artificial heart in Seattle Dentist Barney Clark in 1982 if they had not practiced on neomorts.[13]

Whole brain death proponents claim that slippery slope arguments against brain death are invalid, but brain death opponents assert that acceptance of whole brain death leads one to accepting other looser definitions of death.[14] For if one accepts brain death, one implicitly accepts that certain individuals with integrated spontaneous functioning of major organ systems can be dead. Some brain death criteria permit individuals with integrated spontaneous functioning to be declared dead, and if this can be done, it is not clear why individuals with no responsiveness to their environment cannot also be declared dead.

On the general subject of brain death, James Pallis notes that:

> No culture has ever considered patients in the vegetative state to be dead, or suitable subjects for organ donation. No physician would be authorized anywhere in the world to use the bodies of such patients. . .'certain experimental or instructional purposes'. No doctor would be prepared to perform an autopsy on such a case or to 'initiate burial procedures'.[15]

The success of many organ transplants suggests that the brain dead might not be fully dead, but may still have significant levels of

---

[13] "The Problem of 'Neomorts': Ethicists Confront the Medical Use of Brain-dead Patients" *WP Health*, p. 17, November, 11, 1996. Similar remarks were made by Douglas Walton, *op. cit.* p. 48.

[14] Walton, *op. cit.* P. 2.

[15] See: Lamb, David, *op. cit.* P. 44.

vitality. Many, if not most, organs removed from the brain dead are fully capable of resuming their functioning in other individuals, which suggests that more than pure cellular life is present and that they truly possess integrated spontaneous functioning. They often suffer no significant loss of their functional capability when the whole brain ceases functioning, and they retain their pre-brain death functional capability without any significant limitation. It is not plausible to say that vitality manifested by these organs is the same as is that of the fingernails and hair of the truly deceased. Because many organs function so well when transplanted, it must be affirmed that they display a vitality that is different in kind.

Some authors question whether brain death should be declared for practical ends. Henry Beecher and Isaiah Dorr argue that this is morally legitimate, and Beecher argues that it is immoral and a violation of the dignity of the person to treat a brain dead person as if he or she were alive.[16]

Brain death proponents debate whether brain death is a criterion or a concept of death. It is proposed by many advocates as a criterion and concept of death that compliments the classical criterion of death as the absence of spontaneous integrated respiratory and cardiac function, and this seems to be an accurate assessment.[17] Julius Korein argues that the concept of brain death and criteria of brain death should not be distinguished.[18] He is probably correct, for it seems pretentious to argue that brain death is only a criterion for determining death, for it also seems to define the nature of death as well.

Brain death criteria have been widely accepted in this country as a diagnostic measure for determining full bodily and personal death. However, in Europe, brain death has been accepted primarily for its prognostic power to predict imminent death and

---

[16] Beecher, Henry, K., and Dorr, Isaiah. "The New Definition of Death: Some Opposing Views," *Internationale Zietschrift fur Klinische Pharmakologie, Therapie und Toxicologie*, Vol. 5, (1971) Pp. 120-4.

[17] Walton, *op. cit.* P. 12.

[18] Korein, Julius. "Preface to Brain Death: Interrelated Medical and Social Issues." *Annals of the New York Academy of Sciences*, No. 315 (1978), Pp. 1-10.

not as a diagnostic measure to determine death.[19] In this chapter, this European view will be endorses and new principles for the treatment and care of the brain death will be endorsed. The fundamental reason for supporting this more skeptical view is because of the philosophical problems of brain death and because of the numerous reports of signs of significant vitality among the brain dead.

The nineteenth century was skeptical of medicine's ability to diagnose death, and a similar skepticism is justifiable today because of shifting criteria for determining death and because of the growing number of brain dead patients who show numerous signs of being quite alive.[20] When an organ system ceases integrated spontaneous functioning that might indicate that death is imminent, but it does not necessarily confirm that death has in fact occurred.

In the next part, I wish to point out some of the problems involved in the diagnosis of brain death in order to show that diagnosis of brain death is so unreliable in many circumstances that it should not be used to identify death.

## A
### Determining Whole Brain Death: Problems and Paradoxes

Any attempt to diagnose brain death encounters serious conceptual and practical problems. Various criteria have been proposed to determine when brain death occurs and it is difficult to know which ones, if any, should be adopted. Besides this, there seem to be serious problems with many of these criteria. For example, studies by the American EEG Society in 1970 pointed out that no patient who was diagnosed as brain dead according to EEG

---

[19] See: Doerflinger, Richard. "Resource Paper 'Definition of Death' Legislation", p. 37. Also see: Van Till, Adrienne. "Diagnosis of Death in Comatose Patients Under Resuscitation: A Critical Review of the Harvard Report." *American Journal of Law and Medicine*, Vol. 2, (1976) Pp. 1-40. This British perspective was also noted by the President's Commission for the Study of Ethical Problems in Medicine and Biomedical and Behavioral Research, *Defining Death: Medical, Legal and Ethical Issues in the Determination of Death* (U.S. Government Printing Office, 1981) P. 27.

[20] See: Siegler and Wikler, *op. cit.* P. 1011, and Salamone, *op.cit.*.

standards recovered consciousness.[21] What this study did not mention, however, was that many of these patients may have shown significant signs of vitality after being declared brain dead. The EEG measures the cortex of cerebral hemispheres, and a flat EEG is not necessarily an indicator of loss of vitality. The unreliability of EEG criteria is shown even more clearly by the fact that Harp reported that there have been cases where patients without hypothermia or drug overdose have been certainly diagnosed as being brain dead who have survived despite flat EEG's.[22]

The National Institute of Neurological Diseases and Communicative Disorders and Strokes [NINCDS] issued a set of criteria that demanded that unresponsiveness, loss of spontaneous respiration absence of cephalic responses, flat EEG and no cerebral blood flow to determine the presence of whole brain death. Despite the fact that this is a very strict standard, a survey done of 189 patients showed that some still manifested signs of vitality three months after they were declared brain dead.[23] But Adrienne Van Till has argued that there is much we do not know about the brain because of its complexity, and that diagnosing brain death may not be possible because there might be undetectable vitality at the center of the brain.[24] Henry Veatch implicitly acknowledged the truth of this claim by admitting that brain activity could be present without cerebral activity because the EEG registers only cortical

---

[21] Harp, James, R. "Criteria for the Determination of Death", *Anesthesiology*, Vol. 40, (1974) P. 393. Also, in 1978, the American Neurological Association downgraded EEGs from a requirement for the determination of brain death to an indicator. See: Committee on Irreversible Coma and Brain Death (1978) *Transactions of the American Neurological Association* Vol. 103, P. 320.

[22] *Ibid.* P. 393.

[23] Black, Peter, L. "Definitions of Brain Death" in *Ethical Issues in Death and Dying*. Edited by Tom L. Beauchamp and Seymour Perlin. (Englewood Cliffs: Prentice Hall, 1978) Also see: Walton, Douglas, *op. cit.* P. 19.

[24] Van Till, Adrienne, "How Dead Can You Be? *Medicine, Science and Law*. Vol. 15, (1975) P. 18.

activity.[25] If this is true, it would mean that some patients who meet the NINCDS criteria could in fact still be alive despite the fact that they would be utterly unresponsive.

According to David Lamb, some neuro-scientists acknowledge that the "higher brain" functions such as consciousness and cognition may not be mediated strictly by the cerebral cortex; rather they probably result from complex interrelations between the brainstem and cortex.[26] If these functions interrelate in such a complex fashion, there is sound reason to ask why the other major organ systems and the brain stem do not relate in a similarly complex fashion?

R. B. Shiffer supports the whole brain criterion and suggests that the cardio-respiratory criterion is neither necessary nor sufficient to determine death.[27] He asserts that blood flow, not cardiac or respiratory spontaneity, is crucial for determining death.[28] But blood flow studies can cause serious harm or even death to some patients and using them is an ethically problematic way of determining death.[29] Other techniques to determine brain death can be used such as oxygen consumption, angiography, metabolic techniques and determination of lactic acid in the spinal fluids, but neither is it certain if these can in fact identify actual death and loss of vitality.[30]

The Law Reform Commission of Canada held that the

---

[25] Veatch, Henry. "The Whole-Brain Oriented Concept of Death: An Outmoded Philosophical Formulation." *Journal of Thanatology*, Vol. 3 (1975) Pp. 13-30.

[26] Lamb, David. *Death, Brain Death and Ethics*, (London: Croom Helm, 1984). Pp. 42-3.

[27] Schiffer, R. B., "The Concept of Death: Tradition and Alternative" *Handbook of Electroencephalography and Clinical Neurophysiology* Vol. 12. Edited by Harner, R.N., and Nacquet, R. (Amsterdam: Elsivier, 1974) P. 27.

[28] *Ibid.*

[29] National Institute of Neurological and Communicative Disorders and Stroke, *The NINCDS Collaborative Study of Brain Death* (U.S. Department of Health and Human Services, NIH Publication No. 81-2286: December 1980) Pp. 3, 18-9, 188.

[30] Walton, *op. cit.* Pp. 13-29.

irreversible loss of brain function equalled death, and the enduring loss of spontaneous cardiac and respiratory function accurately indicated brain death.[31] But this criterion raises questions as to whether consciousness or vitality can survive the loss of brain function.

The model statute proposed by the American Bar Association criteria of death virtually ignores the cardiac and respiratory definition of death, and it simply considers death to be equivalent to irreversible cessation of brain function in many instances, but this definition begs a number of questions.[32] What of those cases where basic vital signs remain after loss of brain function? Is it possible for there to be consciousness or perception after the loss of brain function? How does one explain the vitality manifested by many patients who simply loose brain function?

Alex Capron and Leon Kass proposed a definition of death requiring that the uncertain cessation of cardiac or respiratory function be complemented with a certain diagnosis of irreversible cessation of brain function as sufficient for a determination of death.[33] This definition establishes two criteria for death: irreversible loss of spontaneous and integrated cardiac and

---

[31] Law Reform Commission of Canada, *Criteria for the Determination of Death.* Working Paper 23. (Ottawa, 1979).

[32] See: Veith, Frank J.; Fein, Jack M.; Kleiman, Marc A; Tendler, Moses, D; Veatch, Robert M; Kalkines, George. "Brain Death: A status Report of Medical and Ethical Considerations." *Journal of the American Medical Association*, Vol. 238, (1977) P. 1748. This statute holds that "[F]or all legal purposes, a human body with irreversible cessation of total brain function, according to usual and customary standards of medical practice, shall be considered dead."

[33] Capron, Alexander M., and Kass, Leon, R. " A Statutory Definition of the Standards for Determining Human Death." *University of Pennsylvania Law Review*, Vol. 121, (1972). P. 97. Their definition requires the following conditions:

> A person will be considered dead if in the announced opinion of a physician, based on ordinary standards of medical practice, he has experienced an irreversible cessation of spontaneous respiratory and circulatory functions. In the event that artificial means of support preclude a determination that these functions have ceased, a person will be considered dead if in the announced opinion of a physician, based on ordinary standards of medical practice, he has experienced an irreversible cessation of spontaneous brain functions. Death will have occurred at the time when the relevant functions ceased.

respiratory function, and also irreversible loss of brain function. However, we are seeing more cases of patients who have total loss of brain function, as determined by the strictest criteria for death retaining respiratory and cardiac functions for more than just a few hours.[34]

According to Black, widespread brain destruction is found in virtually all cases where brain death has been diagnosed.[35] He and Schwager claim that the brain is necessary for cardiac and respiratory function, and recent developments have indicated that this might not necessarily the case, particularly for short term functioning of these organ systems.[36] We now know that the brain stem functions to moderate and "fine tune" the cardiac and respiratory functions and that these functions can endure without the function of the brain.[37] And even Walton, who accepts brain

---

[34] A BBC *Panorama* program on October 13, 1980 reported the case of four American patients who were diagnosed as brain dead according to various criteria, and it mentioned that there was great pressure on surgeons to diagnose brain death in order to make organs available for transplantation. See: Lamb, David. *op. cit.*, pp. 65-66. Dr. Norman Fost implicitly admitted that many brain dead patients are not fully dead in an editorial:

> A complete summary and refution of the arguments equating brain death with death is beyond the scope of this commentary, but a few observations should be made. Although it is widely accepted that brain death is a valid indicator for discontinuing medical care, the reason is not necessarily because the patient is dead, but because the patient no longer has any interest in being maintained. In this sense, brain death might simply be another in a long list of medical problems which make medical care pointless from the patient's and family's perspective. Other experiences and intuitions suggest that death of the brain is not the same as death in the traditional sense. A headless animal is clearly not dead on that basis alone. We would not feel right about burying someone with a beating heart even though he were brain dead. Brain death appears to be a critical juncture in the complicated process which constitutes death of the organism, but by itself is not equal to death.

[35] Black, Peter. "Brain Death." *New England Journal of Medicine*, Vol. 299, pp. 338-45, 393-401.

[36] Schwager, Robert, L. "Life, Death and the Irreversible Comatose," in *Ethical Issues in Death and Dying*, edited by Tom L. Beauchamp and Seymour Perlin, p. 42. Black, Peter. "Definitions of Brain Death," in *Ethical Issues in Death and Dying*, p. 5.

[37] Doerflinger, "Resource Paper", p. 27.

death criteria, points out that neomort cadavers can be sustained for an extended length of time and their organs can still be implanted in the bodies of others.[38]

Van Till asserts that a patient with no clinical signs might still be alive and be able to experience pain.[39] She argues that simply because a patient does not react physically to pain does not mean that there might not be a physical experience of pain. She notes that the EEG might be able to detect brain function at the periphery of the brain, but not at the center, and that it is possible that there could still be an experience of pain.[40] It is possible that there could be an experience of pain because of the inaccuracy of EEG's.

This view fails to see, however, that death is not dependent on the cessation of brain function or on physical destruction of the brain, but on the cessation of spontaneous of integrated organ system functioning which could mean that death could occur concomitant with loss of brain function. And like others, Veatch recognizes that brain activity could be present without cerebral activity because the EEG only monitors cortical activity.[41] This, of course, means that brain stem activity is not examined and many patients diagnosed as being brain dead could actually be in a persistently vegetative state

Frank Veith *et al.*, argue against whole brain death criteria by arguing that loss of spontaneous respiration must be combined with whole brain death to determine death because a person cannot be considered dead if the person only suffers from paralysis of the motor neurons to the muscles of respiration.[42]

Douglas Walton argues in behalf of the whole brain death criterion in the following way:

---

[38] Walton, *op. cit.* P. 50.

[39] Van Till, Adrienne. "How Dead Can You Be?" P. 18. "[The patient] may simply be incapable of reacting to the stimuli in a manner recognizable to others."

[40] *Ibid.*

[41] Veatch, *op. cit.* Pp. 13-30.

[42] Veith, *et al., op. cit.* P. 1653.

Therefore, because the case for whole-brain death admits of clear, well-established, and widely corroborated criteria, with a clear clinical picture of pathological destruction that irreversibly and inevitably leads to death in a short time, we can see how it is much less open to slippery slope refutions than the case for cerebral death or, indeed, any other current candidate that focuses on one specific part of the brain.[43]

But one must ask Walton if it is so certain that whole brain death does in fact entail loss of vitality or whether it is only a prognosis of imminent death.

He contends that even such reactions as sexual responses in decerebrate cats are not signs of feeling or perception, but it is not so clear that they do not indicate the presence of residual spontaneous functioning of at least some major organ systems?[44] It would seem that they are, and this would suggest that these cats are not fully dead and that they are not utterly devoid of meaningful vitality. Walton believes that these cats have a vestige of life, but what does he mean but this? Does this mean that these creatures must die a second death?

Walton argues that the bodies of the brain dead should be respected as the bodies of other persons.[45] But it is difficult to see why this is morally necessary as the personal dimension of such bodies would be gone after brain death, and it is not clear why the bodies of the brain dead could not be treated as other decerebrate animals are treated. It is not easy to see why their bodies could not be used, as Hans Jonas mentioned, to store tissues, manufacture

---

[43] Walton, *op. cit.* P. 51.

[44] Walton, *op. cit.* Pp. 61-2. Proponents of the cardio-respiratory criterion cite this sort of case to argue that the brain death criterion is insufficient to determine death, and it does suggest that more than just vestigial life remains in the truly brain dead. This sort of response cannot be simply a cellular response, but is in part the result of integrated organic and systemic functioning. It shows even more forcefully what Dr. Fost pointed out that brain death constitutes the final and most tragic trauma to strike a person.

[45] Walton, *op. cit.* Pp. 39, 46.

# MEDICAL ETHICS 215

other tissues or as self-replenishing blood banks.[46]

Walton discusses the capacity for perception as a criterion for death, but he is not sure if its absence should be interpreted as a sign of death because of definitional problems with the notion of perception.[47] He astutely points out that if death is the loss of conscious awareness, experience and perception, then cerebral death should be the criterion for determining death, but doing this would be exceedingly dangerous.[48] He objects to cerebral death criterion for brain death on the basis that one cannot be certain that such individuals are beyond perception. But while virtually the same kinds of questions can be raised about whole brain death, given the fact that not a few of these patients seem to be able to show signs of vitality for an extended period of time. But Walton's objections to cerebral brain death criteria are not based so much on moral concerns as on the difficulty of obtaining a certain diagnosis, and he seems to fail to see the underlying moral issues.

Walton argues further that determination of blood flow is crucial for diagnosis of whole brain death and that our concern should be with the presence of respiration in any form.[49] Apparently contradicting previous statements, he asserts that any sign of respiration is a sign of life.[50] He also affirms Black's contention that the brain is not necessary for cardiac function which implies that respiratory function can also occur where the brain has ceased to function.[51]

Some writers as Dr. Michael Newman, M.D. of St. Boniface

---

[46] Jonas, Hans. "Against the Stream: Comments on the Definition and Redefinition of Death". P. 137.

[47] Walton, op. cit. Pp. 68-69.

[48] Ibid. P. 69.

[49] Walton, op. cit. Pp. 1, 73.

[50] Walton, op. cit. P. 63. "The real point that we should be concerned about is whether there is respiration, but spontaneous or artificial."

[51] Walton, op. cit. P. 64. Also see Black's contentions in "Definitions of Death" in Beauchamp and Perlin, Ethical Issues in Death and Dying. P. 5.

Hospital admit that experiences of pain can exist after mental activity has been lost.[52] He seems to suggest that perceptions of pain and suffering would still be possible in the absence of some critical central nervous system functions.[53] This would seem to argue forcefully against virtually any brain death criterion, as it suggests that perception and experiences of pain are not limited to what can be transmitted by neurological structures. It should also be noted that this possible pain could very well be exceptionally anguishing as the individual experiencing it might not have the intellectual capacity to cope with it.[54] The physical pain of a child is intensified by the fact that it lacks the intellectual and cognitive power to cope with pain and suffering as can the adult. This would seem to suggest that more protective measures should be taken to prevent the brain dead from experiencing pain than should be taken to protect others because of their possible decreased ability to cope with intellectually.

David Lamb defines death as the irreversible loss of function of the "critical organ" of the body and that its irreversible cessation marks the death of the individual.[55] But what precisely is a critical system is not immediately evident. What is it that makes an organ "critical"? Is the critical system that which makes the entire system possible? One wonders if any single organ system is any more critical than any other because of their mutual interdependence. Why are not the cardiac or respiratory systems the critical systems, for they make the operations of the brain stem possible. It would seem that the heart or the lungs would be the critical organ because no other organs can function without air or blood flow, and some other organ systems seem to be able to function rather well without the regulating activity of the brain stem. The brain stem itself may

---

[52] See: Walton, *op. cit.* P. 69.

[53] *Ibid.*

[54] The pain and suffering of the mentally disabled is greater because suffering seems to involve a challenge to the integrity of the self, the ego. Because the disabled often have less ability to maintain the integrity of their egos in the face of the challenges that pain and suffering pose.

[55] Lamb, *op. cit.* Pp. 33-40.

not be replaceable, but it seems that its regulatory function conceivably could be replaced.

## B
## The Concept of Brain Death: Problems and Paradoxes

The concept of brain death, which holds that the person dies with irreversible cessation of the brain, solves many practical problems for some physicians. For by judging the brain dead person to be totally dead, they are free to remove all care and treatments and even transplant organs without any guilt or cooperation in the death of the patient. But just as there is criticism of brain death criteria, so also is there criticism of brain death as a concept of death.

Many accept whole brain death as the death of the person because there is only biological vitality present with no psychological function manifestly present. But proponents of upper brain death argue that the same is the case with the persistently vegetative, and they see no reason why they too should not be called brain dead. Whole brain death proponents criticize cerebral death concepts of death by pointing out that the loss of higher brain function does not predict imminent death, but they fail to see that whole brain death does not predict imminent death infallibly either.[56] This debate is of interest because it suggests that there is a slippery slope involved in acceptance of brain death. The fundamental difficulty with both of these criteria is that they do not explain or account for the presence of vitality that remains in many who suffer either whole or upper brain death .

Adrienne Van Till defends whole brain death concepts of death and claims that a patient ceases to exist and death occurs at this point because there is permanent disintegration of the psychosomatic entity.[57] But one must ask what is meant by the psychosomatic entity? Does this mean that a quadriplegic is not alive because there is no integration between the mind and body of

[56] See: Walton, *op. cit.* P. 41.

[57] Veith, *et al.*, "Brain Death: A Status Report of Medical and Ethical Considerations." P. 1653.

the person? Mental activity does not entail interpersonal communication for Van Till, and she argues that death only truly occurs when whole brain death takes place. We should believe that as long as the physical components necessary for the experience of pain are intact that there can be some psychological experience of pain.

Douglas Walton argues in defense of whole brain death and claims that death should be construed as the cessation of conscious awareness, experience and thinking.[58] One must ask why this is the limit of life and why the loss of all vitality is not the limit? Is this not an excessively disembodied view of death, for it makes bodily existence inherently superfluous? He claims that death is the limit of life as well as the superlimiting possibility of life that enables individuals to transcend life.[59] He argues that this definition of death is justifiable and it makes it possible to rationally explain both brain death and somatic death. Walton argues that loss of whole brain function is a necessary and sufficient condition for death, both as a concept and as a criterion.[60] He rejects loss of perception as a concept of death, and he points out the difficulty in defining perception.[61] But if the experience of pain can be suppressed in an unconscious person, why should not that person be considered dead? Walton admits that some forms of brain stem reflexes could indicate sensations and feelings, but sensations and feelings that could not be interpreted and grasped intellectually, and he denies that they are marks of significant life.[62]

---

[58] See: Walton, *op. cit.* P. 51.

[59] Van Till, "Legal Aspects of the Definition and Diagnosis of Death". *Handbook of Clinical Neurology*. Edited by P. J. Vinken and G. W. Bryun. Vol. 24, No. 2. (Amsterdam and Oxford: North-Holland, 1976.) P. 815.

[60] Walton, *op. cit.* P. 72. "If death is the limit of life, the limit or boundary in question is not the cessation of any functioning of any physical process in the body like respiration or circulation of the blood. It is the limit of conscious awareness, of experience, and of thinking."

[61] *Ibid.* P. 72. Also see: Van Evra, James. "On Death as a Limit". *Analysis.* Vol. 31. (1971) Pp. 170-177.

[62] Walton, *op. cit.* P. 73.

Julius Korein proposes that the brain is irreplaceable and from this he concludes that death equals loss of cerebral function.[63] But, in a certain way, all organs are irreplaceable, and that fact does not make their loss of function equal to death. Even if the brain is irreplaceable, it is not necessarily true that integrated spontaneous functioning of the other organ systems would be lost as well. And Hans Jonas has argued that the very definition of brain death may not be accurate and that we should not be certain that brain dead are truly dead.[64]

Robert Veatch argues that death occurs when there is loss of capacity for social interaction.[65] Some brain death proponents argue that when brain death occurs one has a dead person but a live body.[66] Veith, *et al.* assert that without the brain, the residual activities of organs "do not confer an iota of human personality" on the individual. This would seem to mean that personhood is lodged only in the brain and that the rest of the body is not personal, but is alien to the personal.[67] One must ask what sort of being the post-personal living body is then? Why is it only in the human species that this class transfer occurs shortly before the time of final death?

If this is true it would imply that the persistently vegetative would be dead, and then we would have to ask why do we not bury the comatose and persistently vegetative, or even the severely retarded as they seem to have virtually no capacity for social interaction? Veatch argues for a cerebral concept of brain death because he believes that mental activity is located within the

---

[63] *Ibid.* P. 68.

[64] *Ibid.* Pp. 61-2.

[65] Korein, "Preface to Brain Death: Interrelated Medical and Social Issues." Pp. 1-10.

[66] Jonas, Hans. "Against the Stream: Comments on the Definition and Redefinition of Death," in *Philosophical Essays*. (Englewood Cliffs: Prentice-Hall, 1974.) P. 138.

[67] Veatch, "The Whole-Brain Oriented Concept of Death: An Outmoded Philosophical Formulation". P. 29.

cerebral spheres.[68] Because this is the locus of uniquely human activity, its cessation should mark personal death and the beginning of mere biological life in an individual.

But if it is held that there is not an iota of personhood in an individual who has suffered total loss of brain function then one must face some difficult philosophical problems. The most severe of these is an implied "succession of souls" theory in which the person who is brain dead but somatically alive is not a member of the class of persons, but is a only "somatically alive", a member of the class of animals or "neomorts". This is not only philosophically unacceptable, but it is also biologically unfounded, for there is no indication in nature that the higher mammals engage in "species transfer" when in the process of dying. It also necessitates a double declaration of death, something that has never been seen before in medicine.

Arguments are made that the concept of brain death is a true criterion for death because virtually no one diagnosed as brain dead recovers conscious functioning. This argument misses the crucial point which is that many who are diagnosed as being brain dead show significant signs of life, and this points to a failure in the concept of brain death, and not to just technical misdiagnoses of death. Classical medical theory has applied tutiorist principles to the administration of medical treatments, and one wonders if these principles should not also be applied to the diagnosis and concept of brain death because it is not certain that the brain dead are totally dead. This is so because of the growing number of cases of individuals displaying vital signs after a certain diagnosis of brain death.

## C
### Brain Death and Ensoulment

According to Byrne *et al.*, individuals who have lost brain function should be considered as being in the last stages of dying. When they are in this condition, they should not be subjected to any certainly lethal actions such as removal of their heart or kidneys, even though this does not mean that they must be given aggressive

---

[68] *Ibid.*

medical treatments.[69] This is only one case, but there have been others where those who were purportedly brain dead have shown remarkable signs of vitality. Byrne, *et al.*, argue that the death of an individual is only certain when the physical structures of the brain have been destroyed.[70] When this is verified, the removal of life-sustaining treatments could be permitted. They contend that the death of the person only occurs with certainty when all of the major organ systems have ceased to function.[71] The cessation of function of one major organ system does not always mean that the individual is dead, even though its collapse might trigger the collapse of other organ systems.[72]

Shewmon claims that his doctrines are grounded on Thomistic principles of natural philosophy, and in what follows, these claims will be examined. Shewmon argues that Thomistic natural philosophy supports his claim that those who have suffered loss of neocortical function are dead because he equates absence of the potential for rational operation with the death of the person.[73] Shewmon asserts that the human person is distinguished from the lower animals by intellect and will, and when the neuroanatomical substrata for these are lost then the rational soul ceases to exist. For Shewmon, being born in the human species does not distinguish the human being from animals, for it is the possession of operative rational faculties that differentiates the person from other animals. He affirms that the body is not necessary for the intellectual soul, even though he also asserts that the loss of potential for neocortical functioning necessarily entails the destruction of the rational soul.[74] He does not admit that it is possible that full human nature can remain despite the loss of these operative faculties. He holds that

[69] Byrne and Quay, "Brain Death", P. 461-3.

[70] Byrne and Quay, "Brain Death", *Ibid*. P. 460-61.

[71] Doerflinger, "Resource Paper: Definition of Death Legislation. P. 26.

[72] *Ibid*.

[73] Shewmon, "Brain Death", P. 59.

[74] *Ibid*. Pp. 63-5.

the destruction of the neocortex entails the destruction of the correlative internal senses, but he has not adequately considered the possibility that the soul can remain after these organs cease to function. Shewmon's views of the soul are clearly anti-Cartesian, for he holds that the existence of the soul is in fact totally dependent on the presence of operative capabilities of the body, a notion that has been disputed within the Thomistic tradition.

He admits that the neuroanatomical substrata of the cognitive sense are not known, but he still confidently asserts that the destruction of the cortical spheres destroys the rational soul.[75] He claims this because he believes these structures mediate consciousness, and if they loose their functional potential the intellect, will and rational soul will be destroyed.[76] He argues that the soul is unitary and that there are not three souls in the person, but only one with vegetative, animal and rational functions.[77] But he then declares that it is possible to abolish one function of the soul without destroying the entire soul, which would appear to contradict his claims about the unitary nature of the soul. He affirms that the body is necessary for the soul, but he fails to affirm that the soul can exist when some of the operative functions of the body and soul are lost.[78] Shewmon goes beyond what most reasonable ethicists, courts or Churches would affirm by holding that death occurs when the potential for rational function is lost.[79]

---

[75] *Ibid.* Pp. 56-8.

[76] *Ibid.* P. 54. One must ask if there is any significant behavioral difference between these patients and some other severely handicapped infants who do not have hydroencephalis but who probably will not have the power for rational thought.

[77] *Ibid.* P. 39.

[78] *Ibid.* P. 40.

[79] NCCB "Resource Paper", p. 53. The pro-life committee refused to affirm that the brain dead were certainly and unquestionably dead because of diagnostic problems and problems with the standard itself. They did hold that the brain dead could be considered as being in the final stages of terminal illness and that medical treatments could be removed from them, but they refused to affirm that vital organs could be removed from them simply because they were judged to be "brain dead". P. 51.

He holds that the soul is the substantial form of the body.[80] But he fails to give another account of the nature of the soul, which is that it is the first act of the body, the principle of the person.[81] As the substantial form of the person, he believes that it can only come in to existence when matter is properly prepared to receive it.[82] On this account, the rational soul could only begin to exist at the end of the third month of gestation. He proposes an unduly narrow definition of the human soul and he ignores other aspects and functions of the soul. The soul is the first or vivifying substantial act of the body and its operations are its second acts.[83] It is the first act of the body and is not an operative potency. But the soul itself is the independent first act of these operations which are its second acts.[84] The soul is a causally complex form which prepares matter for its operations, and it contains the vegetative, sentient and rational faculties within itself.[85] The soul is the first act of the human body, and is the formal, final and efficient cause of the person.[86] It is the principle of vital operations and of the perfections required for matter to exercise its operations.

A fundamental problem with Shewmon's theories about individuals who loose cortical function is that they have to engage in some sort of "species transfer", moving from the class of human beings to the class of "humanoid animals", when they die, and the biological evidence that this occurs is almost nonexistent.[87] Rather

---

[80] Aquinas, Thomas. *In II De Anima*, n. 233.

[81] Klubertanz, S.J. George, Peter. *The Philosophy of Human Nature.* (New York: Appleton-Century-Crofts, 1953) P. 313.

[82] Gerber, Rudolf. "When is the Human Soul Infused?" *Laval Theologique y Philosophique*, 1966, Vol. 22, No. 2, p. 244.

[83] *Ibid*. P. 244.

[84] *Ibid*. P. 244.

[85] *Ibid*. P. 244.

[86] *Ibid*. P. 243.

[87] See Chapter One.

than being subhuman beings, it seems that the brain dead, permanently unconscious, comatose and demented are still human beings, but human beings with a minimal level of intellectual functioning, not unlike infants. These individuals may be debilitated and incapable of intellectual functioning, but they are still human beings and members of the human species.

Shewmon mistakenly assumes that it is impossible for the rational soul to be present if there is no power to perform rational operations.[88] He holds that the existence of rational soul requires the existence of organs capable of these operations. The functional integrity of the tertiary association cortices determines if the rational soul can exist or not.[89] This is only a speculative opinion, however, for one cannot identify the soul with either the bodily organs themselves or with the functions of the organs. He fails to see that the absence of the power to exercise reason does not entail the nonexistence of the rational soul.[90] It is quite possible that the rational soul could exist even when the power to exercise rational functions was lost.[91] It is only a matter of conjecture that the soul is not present when its powers cannot be exercised. It is not certain that the soul ceases to exist when rational function is lost, and unless there is conclusive proof to the contrary, individuals without cortical function must be treated in practice as if it had a rational soul.

He claims that consciousness can be sustained and continued by electrical stimulation of the midbrain.[92] However, it is merely a speculative and hypothetical opinion that the midbrain can function fully and completely in isolation from the other organs. That all conscious thought comes from the midbrain is probably true, but that does not mean that individuals without midbrain function are not persons in the full sense. He claims that proper functioning of

---

[88] Shewmon, "Brain Death", p. 49.

[89] Shewmon, "Brain Death", p. 57.

[90] Ibid. P. 243.

[91] Gerber, "Infused", P. 243.

[92] Shewmon, "Brain Dead", P. 250.

the organs is required for the presence of the soul, and holds that the destruction of these organs would bring about the destruction of the soul. When there is the loss of the functional anatomical reserve, then there is a substantial change in the person and the rational soul is destroyed.[93]

Shewmon's ideas are not new. In 1973 Robert Rizzo and Paul Yonder made virtually the same arguments.[94] And probably the best response to these claims has been made by Benedict Ashley and Kevin O'Rourke:

> First, the radical structures necessary and sufficient to constitute the unified organism of the human person would have to be found in the human brain separated from the rest of the body. This certainly is plausible from what is now known. Second, most of the brain would have to be considered unnecessary for the specifically human functions of thinking and willing, but existing only to maintain and move the body and supply the higher brain centers with nourishing materials. This also is plausible, but the present state of knowledge on this is far from certain. It is generally recognized today that the brain is a system of subsystems which are intimately interdependent. Although it is possible to localize such functions as speech and sight in particular parts of the brain, this is no proof that only one such part is involved in the function or even that it is its primary center. since inhibition of a merely secondary or auxiliary part of a system may impede its function. Third, if it were certain that these higher centers are sufficient for the radical unity of the human organism, it would be very difficult to determine their exact condition without an autopsy. The mere absence of function would not establish their condition. Perhaps someday, it may be possible to determine when in special cases such centers are totally

---

[93] *Ibid.* P. 62.

[94] Rizzo, Robert, and Yonder, Paul. "Definition and Criteria of Clinical Death", *Linacre Quarterly*, 1973, Vol. 40, pp. 223-233.

destroyed, but at present this is not the case.[95]

Shewmon's views concerning the presence of the soul affirm the outmoded doctrine of succession of souls. During the dying process he implies that the rational soul is the first to be destroyed, and only after that are the animal and vegetative souls destroyed. Events of this nature could only occur if a succession of souls occurred during human ontogenesis, which he denies takes place. In Aquinas' time there was some scientific basis for the succession of souls theory, but contemporary scientific evidence for this theory is not without dispute.

Shewmon says that he only wants those who have lost cortical function to be treated as if they were dead, but he states elsewhere that they are actually dead.[96] If the latter is true, then these persons actually suffer two deaths. They die once when they loose the substrata for intellect and will and they die again when they are brought to physiological death by dehydration, starvation or lethal injection. In our contemporary philosophical climate, it is hard to accept these views for they seem to be arguments more of convenience than of sound philosophical analysis.

## D
## Care and Brain Death

When facing the problem of diagnosing states of permanent coma or persistent vegetative state, Shewmon explicitly admits that the medical causes of many forms of persistent unconsciousness are not known.[97] What he failed to mention is that ordinarily the primary difference between the comatose and permanently

---

[95] Ashley, Benedict; and O'Rourke, Kevin. *Health Care Ethics*, Second Edition. (St. Louis, Mo: The Catholic Hospital Association, 1982) pp. 368-9.

[96] Shewmon, "Brain Death", p. 80. In this passage, Shewmon calls on society to treat the permanently comatose, demented and hydroencephalic as dead. But two sentences later, he refers to them as cadavers.

[97] *Ibid.* P. 80.

vegetative is a statistical difference.[98] He argues that the use of EEG's and CT scans can certainly determine the complete loss of cortical function, yet experts have pointed out that these procedures cannot always detect neuronal activity at the very center and core of the brain.[99] In the persistently unconscious and comatose, there is clearly some form of human life present, but it is just not clear at the present time what kind of life this is. Because of this uncertainty, responsible moral action would require that the life these individuals be treated as human beings with a full compliment of human and moral rights. He reduces the life of these individuals, however, to purely animal life when it is by no means certain that this is true.

In his discussion of the status of the seriously demented, he contends that they do not have rational souls because their level of intellectual functioning is not compatible with the human essence.[100] He actually holds that the demented are without a spiritual soul and that they are in the next life even though their bodies remain on earth in the form of a "humanoid animal".[101] He claims these individuals lack a rational soul despite the fact that their neocortical spheres have not been destroyed and they only suffer from diminished neocortical functioning. Even though they can experience pain and suffer only from diminished neocortical functioning, he asserts that they are not persons and that their bodies are incompatible with the human essence.

He does note, however, that it is very difficult to diagnose

---

[98] *Ibid.* P. 70.

[99] See: NCCB "Resource Paper", p. 38. Van Till has argued that the only certain test for death of the brain is that which demonstrates that there is no blood flow to the brain, something which EEG's are unable to determine with certainty. She recommends angiography as the only certain direct test for the death of the brain. And a study done by the National Institute of Neurological and Communicative Disorders and Stroke found that neither the Harvard criteria nor other brain death criteria were found to be consistently correlated with evidence of brain destruction. See: *The NINCDS Collaborative Study of Brain Death*. (U.S. Department of Health and Human Services, NIH Publication No. 81-2286, Dec. 1980).

[100] *Ibid.* P. 60.

[101] *Ibid.* P. 60.

dementia and that it is not known what neuro-anatomical substrata are necessary for rational thought and the presence of the will and intellect.[102] Dementia develops in stages, and Shewmon admits that the precise point at which the neurological substrata of the intellect and will are destroyed cannot be known.[103] But he does claim that there is a critical point somewhere at which potential for cortical function is destroyed, and this gives a general justification for bringing these patients to death by dehydration or starvation.[104] One wonders why he does not apply this criterion to the severely retarded because they have a level of functioning that is lower than some demented and should therefore not be considered as having a rational soul either. However, he does not appear to want to admit that his principles justify deliberate killing of even mildly handicapped newborns. Shewmon goes far beyond what most responsible ethicists and physicians would hold about the status of these individuals. For, he seems convinced that the demented should not be given care or support and that "medical games" should not be played with these patients.[105]

Shewmon also claims that hydroencephalic newborns do not have rational souls because there can be no development of the cerebral cortices in these children.[106] It is probably true that they do not have the capacity for rational thought and never will, but Shewmon excludes them from all membership in the human species precisely because of this condition. Contrary to what he asserts, they may not be capable of consciousness, but they still possess a human nature as they are born in the human species, and like other human beings, they retain their moral right not to be directly killed and have their lives deliberately destroyed.

Shewmon believes that traditional Catholic baptismal practice endorses his views that hydroencephalic infants lack a

---

[102] *Ibid.* P. 54, 57.

[103] *Ibid.* P. 59-60.

[104] *Ibid.* P. 78-9.

[105] *Ibid.* P. 80.

[106] *Ibid.* Pp. 72-3.

rational soul because conditional baptism was only given when monsters were born with two chests and one head or to the second head of a child born with one chest and two heads.[107] Rather than justifying his claims, however, this practice supports the presumption that a rational soul could be present even in the severely malformed. This practice affirmed the view that the safer course of moral action should be taken in practice when dealing with such individuals and that there should be very limited presumptions of nonpersonhood if a child is biologically abnormal.

His views about the conditions under which the soul is present are doubtfully in accord with the teachings of Aquinas, and certainly not in accord with the teachings of the Church. Pius XII held that death could not be diagnosed with certainty until all of the vital functions had ceased.[108] He is even quite far beyond the AMA or any court judgment that has yet been handed down in our nation.[109] And not even the President's Commission for the Study of Ethical Problems in Medicine and Biomedical and Behavioral Research would endorse Shewmon's proposal that the permanently unconscious and demented could be brought to death by starvation, dehydration or lethal injection, and yet Shewmon holds all of these out as possibilities.[110]

Shewmon has not proved his case that there is certainly not a rational soul in the individuals he describes, and as we shall see that this calls into question his ethical prescriptions.

[107] *Ibid.* P. 47.

[108] NCCB, "Resource Paper", pp. 51-3.

[109] *Opinions of the Judiciary Council of the American Medical Association*, 1984, para. 2.11.

[110] President's Commission for the Study of Ethical Problems in Medicine and Biomedical and Behavioral Research, *Deciding to Forego Life-Sustaining Treatment: Ethical, Medical and Legal Issues in Treatment Decisions*. (Washington, D.C: U.S. Government Printing Office, 1983.) P. 190 The Commission allowed removal of food and fluids from the comatose when these were judged to be of no benefit, however this sort of decision could be made, but it did not allow giving lethal injections to individuals, not did it include the demented in the category of those who could be denied nutrition and hydration. It also failed to assert that these individuals were not persons or lacked a rational soul.

Dr. Shewmon shows a great deal of familiarity with Thomistic natural philosophy, but he apparently accepts neither the classical moral theory of Thomas nor the classical medical distinction between normal care and medical treatments. One cannot dispute the assertion that some forms of medical treatments can be removed from the brain dead, and some patients who have lost neocortical function. But one must take issue with his assertion that all nutrition and fluids can be withdrawn from these individuals, or that lethal injections be given because these individuals are "humanoid animals". To do any of these risks or certainly involves direct killing, and at least according to the classical moral tradition, and are therefore impermissible.

Contrary to what he claims, it seems that life-sustaining nutrition and fluids should be given to those diagnosed as "brain dead" who display significant signs of vitality with minimal levels of assistance. Because it seems that some "brain dead" patients can sustain significant signs of vitality with this assistance, readily providable nutrition and fluids that can be given through basic nursing care procedures should be given to them. If patients in the conditions Shewmon describes are beyond pain and cannot suffer anymore, then no harm is done by providing them with food and fluids. And if they can still experience pain, then denying them food and fluids is a great good for them, as this prevents the individual from experiencing the agony of starvation or dehydration.

Shewmon has ignored the critical principle of medical practice which holds that the more protective course of action is followed when there is a risk that innocent human life would be deliberately destroyed.[111] Shewmon proposes that certainly lethal action be taken with various classes of patients because he refuses to admit that they are bearers of moral rights. Believing that these individuals do not possess any moral rights, he denies that the more protective course is to be followed with them. In this respect, he

---

[111] See: O'Donnell, S.J., Thomas. *Medicine and Christian Morality*. (New York: Alba House, 1976) P. 17. O'Donnell points out that where there are positive doubts about the morality of an action that the safer course of action is to be followed, which is a classical principle of probabilism. In the cases discussed by Shewmon, there is positive doubt as to whether removal of nutrition and fluids is culpably lethal because it is not certain what kind of human life is present in the brain dead, persistently unconscious, demented and hydroencephalic.

stands more in the modern than in the classical tradition, for modern thought ascribes rights to individuals because they display the traits of psychological personhood rather than on account of their human nature. These tendencies have been denied by the natural law tradition, however, and this tradition holds that rights are possessed by human beings because they had a spiritual, human nature, and not because they had the psychological traits of personhood.[112] To be fully in accord with the natural philosophical and metaphysical thought of Aquinas, Shewmon should hold that the certain possession of personhood in the psychological sense is not necessary for the ascription of human and natural moral rights, and that these rights should be ascribed to those born in the human species.

Shewmon does not seem to believe that any moral culpability attaches to actions which directly intend the death of others either by commission or omission. For once a judgment has been made that the rational soul is no longer present, no matter how unsound that judgment might be, he holds that there is nothing immoral in willing death by either positive acts or omissions. Shewmon implies that the moral duty to refrain from directly lethal actions is overridden or nonexistent when certain medical conditions obtain. What this indicates is that his moral theory is not within the classical Catholic moral tradition, but is fundamentally a "quality of life" medical ethic, for he holds that when mental capacities deteriorate to an unspecified point that there are neither duties to provide treatment and care, nor duties to refrain from directly and positively lethal actions.

Shewmon believes that it is legitimate for the physician to deliberately, positively and intentionally bring death to patients for a variety of reasons, and he does not consider these actions to be culpably direct killing.[113] He provides no solid and persuasive reasons to show why giving lethal injections to patients is not direct killing and he only says that they are permissible when there are

---

[112] Finnis, John. *Natural Law and Natural Rights*. (New York: Oxford University Press, 1980.) Pp. 223-226. Finnis argues that such rights as the absolute right not to be tortured is possessed by individuals in virtue of their humanity and not because of any grant given by individuals, governments or societies.

[113] Shewmon, "Brain Death", pp. 78-9.

sufficient reasons. By never stating what these sufficient reasons might be, he establishes a purely formal moral standard for giving medically vulnerable patients lethal injections which is quite dangerous. Bringing death by lethal injections is never a morally permissible course of action, as this is a positive, direct, lethal act that is never morally choice worthy.

Shewmon is concerned that intensive care units not be populated with demented, brain dead, comatose or permanently unconscious patients, and he seems to want to banish them from our health care institutions. He is tired of "playing medical games" with these patients he calls cadavers.[114] While he retains Thomistic natural law principles to verify his claims that the soul is not present in the permanently comatose, he rejects the moral principles which Thomas employs to regulate actions directed at these individuals. He is quite willing to abandon Thomistic moral principles and argue that culpable omissions and positive lethal acts are not only morally tolerable but mandatory in some instances to clean out intensive care units. All of these are proposed on the speculative and probable opinion that human beings who have lost the power to exercise rational functions are no longer in possession of a moral right not to be directly killed. Because Shewmon has failed to acknowledge that opinions concerning the presence of the rational soul are entirely speculative and therefore not binding on ethical decision making, he has failed to prove his case that the actions he proposes can be taken against the brain dead, permanently unconscious, comatose and severely handicapped.

Dr. Shewmon's article should be taken very seriously, for he is denying the very personhood of the demented, permanently unconscious and comatose, and his language indicates a clear bias against these individuals. He is a leading figure in American medicine, and his attitudes should persuade us that the medically vulnerable are in imminent danger of becoming medical hostages whose lives and vitality is wholly dependent on the good will and compassion of caregivers and not on strict standards of medical care and treatment.

## CONCLUSION

---

[114] *Ibid.* P. 80.

Advocates of whole brain death and cerebral brain death fail to see that death occurs when the spontaneous functioning of the major organ systems ceases irreversibly. Because of all of the conceptual and technical problems with the diagnosis and definition of brain death, it seems morally imperative to refrain from any deliberately lethal omissions or commissions with those diagnosed as or suspected to be brain dead as long as signs of integrated organ functioning remain present.

I suggest that those who have suffered total and irreversible loss of whole brain function but who manifest signs of vitality through integrated spontaneous organic and systemic functioning should be given at least normal care, even though medical and therapeutic treatments can be withdrawn. Because there are solid grounds for believing that not all brain dead individuals are truly dead, I urge that the brain dead be given nutrition and hydration, sanitary care and protection from exposure when they show significant signs of vitality. In addition, I do not believe that vital organs should be removed from them as long as they show these significant signs of vitality.

And even further, I would suggest that the only proper moral course of action to take with the brain dead who show significant signs of vitality is to refrain from taking directly and certainly lethal actions against them, actions such as removal of vital organs or administration of lethal injections. Where brain death has been diagnosed and there are signs of extended integrated spontaneous functioning, routine nursing care, respiratory and cardiac support should be given.

Douglas Walton commented that arguments for and against brain death have an "open texture" and a continually changing aspect that leads to inconclusiveness, and he counsels against taking pessimistic approaches in reflections about the definition and diagnosis of brain death.[115] Yet in the face of this inconclusiveness and ambiguity, as admitted by a strong and learned proponent of brain death, criteria, it seems that skepticism and reticence is a proper approach to brain death criteria and diagnoses. This skepticism does not flow from intellectual malice but from what

---

[115] Walton, *op. cit.* P. 83

appear to be fundamental flaws in these criteria and concepts. A skeptical and conservative attitude toward claims that those who have lost whole brain function are fully dead is not unjustified in the face of profoundly problematic and unproven hypotheses. And the moral consequences of this skepticism be translated into a morally protective course of action.

# CHAPTER NINE
# THE JURISPRUDENCE OF ASSISTED FEEDING

The aim of the international mercy killing movement has been to gain legal and social endorsement of mercy killing by first gaining legal and social endorsement of euthanasia by omission of food and water, and then to gain endorsement for active mercy killing by means of lethal injection. Because of the emergence of this movement, the need has arisen to develop legislation to prevent suicide among the medically vulnerable and protect them from medical abuse and neglect. To facilitate this legislation, it is necessary to develop a theoretical understanding of the nature of assisted feeding, and a set of ethical criteria for their administration that will justify making their provision legally mandatory in specific instances.

In this chapter, I will discuss some current theories of the nature of nutrition and fluids and principles that should govern their provision to show that the theories proposed fail to provide an adequate moral basis for laws that would forbid discriminatory withdrawal of food and fluids from medically dependent and vulnerable adults. The question of the precise nature of assisted feeding and nutrition has been considered recently by a number of philosophers, moralists and courts. No consensus has been reached on this issue, despite, despite the claims of some that one is developing, and courts are divided on the nature and legal obligations to feed various classes of patients.

The last chapter of this book will discuss the principles of jurisprudence that can be employed to justify such legislation. But what is lacking at the present time is an ethical theory that can justify these laws and jurisprudential principles. I will also suggest in this chapter that the only way in which laws requiring that individuals not be denied food and water on a discriminatory basis is by holding that its provision is an aspect of normal care in some cases. I will argue that this understanding is the only one that can adequately stand as a criterion for such laws. In what follows, I will also try to show that assisted feeding cannot be compared to medical treatments in an unqualified manner, and that there are such significant differences between feeding by IV and NG tube and the use of a respirator that this comparison can be called into question.

To do this, I will first summarize the recent thought of some leading moralists to determine if their understanding of the nature of assisted feeding and the ethical principles that govern its provision can support legislation to protect the medically vulnerable. Then I will argue that only by considering it to be normal care can this be done. The moralists who will be considered are Fr. John Paris, S.J., Fr. Richard McCormick, S.J., Fr. John Connery, S.J., Fr. Thomas O'Donnell, S.J., Dr. William May, Fr. Edward Bayer, Dr. Daniel Callahan and Dr. Germain Grisez. To show that this is the only way of doing this I will show how assisted feeding differs from medical treatments and respirators in particular.

## A
## FEEDING PATIENTS: ETHICAL AND LEGAL OPINIONS

### 1
### John Paris, S.J.

Fr. John Paris, S.J., has been very active in expressing his views on the issue of providing assisted feeding, and in the *Barber* case he testified that it was no different from other medical treatments.[1] Because they were no different, he held that they should only be provided when they were of benefit to the patient, when the patient could be expected to gain some neurological recovery from their provision.[2] Fr. Paris holds that "assisted feeding" is only a beneficial medical treatment when there is a prognosis of neurological recovery for the patient who receives it.[3] But what this means is not clear. Would it mean that Hector Rodas

---

[1] Paris, S. J., John, J., and McCormick, S. J., Richard. "The Catholic Tradition on the Use of Nutrition and Fluids", *America*. May 2, 1987, P. 358.

[2] In reporting the decision of the New Jersey Supreme Court's decision *in re Conroy*, Fr. Paris reported without comment and apparently favorably that "artificial feeding, like any other medical treatment, may with procedural safeguards,. be withheld or withdrawn from an incompetent patient if it proves disproportionately burdensome and contrary to the patient's values or interests." See: Paris, S.J., John, J; and Reardon, J.D., Frank, E. "Court Responses to Withholding or Withdrawing Artificial Nutrition and Fluids", *Journal of the American Medical Association*, (Vol. 253, No. 15., P. 2245.

[3] *Barber v. People*, 147 Cal. App. 3d 1006, 195 Cal. Rptr. at 490.

was morally justified in starving himself to death because he had no prognosis of recovery? What exactly constitutes recovery? One must also ask if he is not placing too much weight on some of the secondary and peripheral consequences of feeding, for we do not ordinarily demand that feeding enhance our neurological functioning before receiving it. Usually we take food and water because they meet our nutritional and hydrational needs, and if they promote our neurological functioning, that is well and nice, but if they fail to do this, that does not make their consumption illegitimate.

Fr. Paris apparently considers all actions which health care professionals perform for patients or which maintain medically stable patients to be medical treatments because they are given under their orders, and he makes no distinction between care, ordinary medical treatment and extraordinary medical treatments. Fr. Paris has never shown how nutrition and fluids actually cure, remedy and palliate clinical conditions or why they are not aspects of normal, routine, customary and ordinary nursing care that is to be provided to patients who need it. Fr. Paris' views are essentially discriminatory against the handicapped because they demand that food and fluids be of benefit to a patient which is not required for others to be given food and fluids.

Fr. Paris' account of the conditions under which nutrition and fluids can be required cannot stand as an ethical basis for laws designed to protect the medically vulnerable because his theory is frankly discriminatory against individuals with certain kinds of disabilities. Discrimination occurs when an individual is denied a benefit that can be equally enjoyed by one individual as well as others because of some condition that is extraneous to the individuals or the benefit under consideration. It was thus discriminatory to deny blacks equal access to educational opportunities as they could enjoy the benefits as of this opportunity as much as could others. Similarly, denying successful and readily providable nutrition and fluids to medically stable patients is discriminatory because they can enjoy the same substantial benefits of food and water as can those to those who have no neurological impairments. Food and water sustain the lives of both the neurologically impaired and those without neurological impairments. In addition, their denial equally and certainly brings death to both classes. Fr. Paris' criteria for providing nutrition and fluids, therefore, cannot be accepted as an adequate standard for developing law to protect the medically vulnerable.

## 2
## Richard McCormick, S.J.

Fr. Richard McCormick, S.J., objected to the brief submitted by the New Jersey Catholic Conference in the Nancy Ellen Jobes case and he argued that the Catholic tradition considered assisted feeding to be a medical treatment.[4] It is ironic to find Fr. McCormick arguing for a position by invoking the orthodox tradition because he has been a major revisionist of that tradition and very critical of it since *Humanae Vitae*. But conceiving of it as a medical treatment means that it can be withdrawn when there is no potentiality for relationality in the person receiving it. To be consistent with his previous positions, he would have to argue that the "quality of life" of the person receiving it would have to warrant its provision.[5]

Fr. McCormick invokes the Catholic medical-ethical tradition to justify his view of the nature of assisted feeding, but he misapplies most of the criteria that have traditionally been used to administer it.[6] For example, the tradition would focus on what the treatment did rather than on the quality of life that was brought about by its provision as does McCormick, but he does not accept this. The tradition also developed its distinctions, not so much to protect patients from overtreatment as to protect them from undertreatment. Rather than facilitating protection of the medically

---

[4] Paris, S.J., John.; and McCormick, S.J., Richard. "The Catholic Tradition on the Use of Nutrition and Fluids", pp. 356-9.

[5] For a perspective representative of his "quality of life ethic" see his: "To Save or Let Die", *America*, July 14, 1974, and his "Caring or Starving? The Case of Claire Conroy." *America*, April 6, 1986, Pp. 269-273.

[6] *Ibid.* For example, he invokes Fr. Gerald Kelly's principles but he fails to see that Kelly's principles applied to a *terminally ill* unconscious patient who would die shortly even if feeding were to be provided. However, in he cases he discusses, the patients such as Paul Brophy, Clarence Herbert and Nancy Ellen Jobes, the patients were not terminal. The crisis presented in these cases resulted from the fact that they were not going to die soon and not that they were going to die quickly. It was the latter sort of case which Fr. Kelly addressed, and not the former.

undertreatment. Rather than facilitating protection of the medically vulnerable, Fr. McCormick's understanding would facilitate denying them food and water because of their purported lack of relationality potentiality.

Like the position adopted by Fr. Paris, Fr. McCormick's cannot stand as an adequate criterion for legislation to protect the medically vulnerable from discriminatory withdrawal of food and water because it is biased against those with handicapped communication or relational abilities. Nutrition and hydration have the same effect on those who cannot "relate" to others as it has on those with these abilities, and there is no good reason to deny it to those who can live with its provision. To deny them nutrition and fluids because they lack these abilities is an unethical and discriminatory denial of a benefit based on a condition for which they are not responsible. The category of patients lacking "relational potentiality" is so ambiguous and ill-defined that it has the power to deny basic and minimal care for a wide variety of individuals. It is so difficult to determine who actually is a member of this class that an untold number of disabled persons could be denied food and water that could significantly sustain their lives.

### 3
### John Connery, S.J.

Fr. John Connery, S.J., suggests that assisted feeding is a combination of normal eating and drinking and of a medical treatment. Unlike Fr. Paris and Fr. McCormick, however, he holds that there are many more circumstances in which assisted feeding should be provided than in which medical treatments should be given.[7] Against the opinions of Fr. Paris and McCormick, he objected to the removal of food and water from Clarence Herbert, Claire Conroy, Paul Brophy and Nancy Ellen Jobes.[8] Fr. Connery

---

[7] Connery, S.J., John. "The Ethics of Withholding/Withdrawing Nutrition and Hydration" *The Linacre Quarterly*, February 1987, Vol. 54, No. 1, P. 98.

[8] Connery, S.J., John. "In the Matter of Clare Conroy", *The Linacre Quarterly*, November 1985, Vol. 52, No 4. Pp. 321-334. Also See: Connery, S.J., John. "The Withdrawal of Mr. Herbert's Feeding Tube: Was It Justified?" *Hospital Progress*. February, 1984, Pp. 32-35, 70.

denies that there are any plausible circumstances in which the burden to society or the scarcity of resources could justify removal of feeding from patients.[9] He does admit that in the speculative order a patient could omit assisted feeding if it caused grave financial burdens to one's family.[10] He also admits that assisted feeding could be withdrawn or withheld if it could not appreciably prolong life.[11] In saying this, he separates himself from the thought of Frs. McCormick and Paris who hold that there must be some prospect for neurological recovery and he does not require that there be such an effect of feeding for it to be obligatory.[12]

Fr. Connery has also argued that feeding could be removed or rejected by a patient when judged to be *very* burdensome.[13] He argues strongly against providing food and water according to quality of life criteria and he warns that adopting these criteria could rapidly result in uncontrolled denial of food and water from medically vulnerable patients.[14] He makes clear distinctions between intending death through the withholding or withdrawal of feeding and permitting or allowing it legitimately by not providing what is truly burdensome.[15] He also admits that the long-term use of assisted feeding could make it radically burdensome, and therefore

---

[9] Fr. Connery holds that the differences between assisted feeding and other medical treatments are not morally relevant and that the same conditions that apply to the administration of medical treatments should govern the provision of food and water. See: "The Ethics of Withdrawing/Withholding Nutrition and Fluids", P. 19.

[10] *Ibid*. P. 21.

[11] *Ibid*. P. 20

[12] *Ibid*. Pp. 24-5. Connery objects to withdrawal of food and water from persistently vegetative patients simply because they are in this condition. Frs. Paris and McCormick seem to want to withdraw their food and water precisely because they are in this condition.

[13] Connery,S.J., John. "In the Matter of Claire Conroy", P. 328.

[14] Connery,S.J., John. "The Ethics of Withdrawing/Withholding Nutrition and Hydration", Pp. 22-3.

[15] *Ibid*. P. 25.

Fr. Connery rightly admits that the law should not permit withdrawal or withholding of assisted feeding on the basis of quality of life judgments because this could result in loss of control. However, he does not seem to see that allowing withdrawal or withholding of feeding because of judgments that it would be too burdensome to the patient or family could have the same result. To prevent this from occurring, it is necessary that a different moral standard be developed that would prevent loss of control.

Fr. Connery's criteria are more suited to development of laws protecting the medically vulnerable and dependent than are those of Fr. Paris or Fr. McCormick, but it is not clear that his claim that the long-term use of assisted feeding is not an obligatory procedure would not be not discriminatory against those with enduring or permanent disabilities. It is not clear that this ethical principle could stand as an ethical foundation for laws the protect the disabled and handicapped from discriminatory removal of food and water. And it is not immediately evident that Fr. Connery's strict criteria for the withdrawal or withholding of nutrition and fluids can be fully harmonized with the traditional teachings of the Church on the provision of medical treatments.

Long-term use of nutrition and fluids brings the same benefit for patients that short-term use does, which is to sustain the life of the individual, and this benefit does not diminish with time. The effect and withdrawal of food and water provided patients over the long-term is the same as on those receiving it only for the short term: certain death. And even if assisted feeding is given for an extended length of time, the amount of labor involved is so much greater that it makes it radically burdensome for the provider.

To argue that assisted feeding can become burdensome over the long term could be dangerous because that principle could commit one to accepting the radical burdensomeness of long term but successful insulin injections, use of wheelchairs, walkers or other such devices, for example. Young nursing home patients could be denied minimal care because of claims of health care providers or family members that their care was too burdensome. For these patients, it would seem that Fr. Connery's criteria would be discriminatory. And, it is also to be feared that his criteria permitting rejection of long-term assisted feeding might put the category of permanently incompetent patients such as Nancy Ellen Jobes at even risk. A further difficulty with his theory is that the law could not distinguish between long-term and short-term use in a way that would not be wholly arbitrary and discriminatory.

None of this should be interpreted to imply that Fr. Connery's theory is necessarily erroneous, but only that it cannot be translated into a nondiscriminatory and nonarbitrary legal norm in its present state. It may be impeccable moral theory, but it is doubtful that it could stand as a basis for protective legislation on this matter.

### 4
### Thomas O'Donnell, S.J.

Fr. Thomas O'Donnell, S.J., has argued that feeding is useless when it is provided to a definitely unconscious and terminally ill patient who cannot "use" the good of life that is sustained by feeding.[16] He holds that "terminal unconsciousness" makes feeding extraordinary.

> I also contend in the case of terminal unconsciousness, artificial feeding can become an extraordinary means of what (as noted above) Father Gerald Kelly called the "mere prolonging of life" under an intolerable burden (even financial) to others and perhaps also under the rubric of clinically useless.[17]

Fr. O'Donnell claims elsewhere that feeding can be withheld or withdrawn when their burdens are judged to be excessive. He states that:

> Subject to any subsequent teaching of the Holy See, we would hold that, at least in the case of incurable pathology accompanied by definitely established irreversible coma and the attendant inability to take

---

[16] O'Donnell, S.J., Thomas. "Fr. O'Donnell Responds". *The Medical Moral Newsletter*, Vol. 24, No. 4, April 1987. P. 16.

[17] *Ibid.* P. 16.

food and water normally, artificial nutrition and hydration could be withheld or withdrawn either because the burden of continuing treatment would be disproportionate to the benefit, or because their continuation would be judged not to be clinically significant or therapeutic.[18]

One must wonder if this principle is adequate for providing assisted feeding, for it would seem that there are treatments or forms of care such hygienic care or protection from exposure that could be given to the terminally unconscious which are no more burdensome than assisted feeding that cannot be ethically withdrawn. Would Fr. O'Donnell agree that these could be withheld from the terminally unconscious because they too cannot be "used" by these patients? Why could not these principles be applied to the terminal demented or profoundly mentally ill, as they seem to be able to make "use" out of assisted feeding as much as could the terminally unconscious? Fr. O'Donnell's principles seem to be so loose that they could pose serious threats to the mentally and emotionally disabled.

Fr. O'Donnell argues that removing food and water to cause death is different from removing it when it is the occasion of the death of the patient.[19] This is an excellent distinction that has been incorporated into the American legal tradition which recognizes that a man who suffered severe brain damage after being shot was killed by the gunman and not by the physician who later removed the respirator and life-support systems.[20] The physician's action was not the cause of death but was merely the occasion on which death that was inflicted by the gunman occurred.

This distinction is quite valuable, but it must be applied with great care. While the law acknowledges this distinction, it should be applied in the way it is applied for the administration of urinary

---

[18] Comment" *Medical-Moral Newsletter*, Vol. 24, No 2, February 1987, P. 7.

[19] *Ibid.*

[20] See: Stanley, Lisa. "The Law of Homicide: Does it Require a Definition of Death?", *Wake Forest Law Review*, Vol. 11, (1975),pp. 253-255.

catheters or insulin. With these forms of treatment, the law requires them to be provided to a "medically stable" for whom they are successful. Just as the law would consider withdrawing insulin or a successful urinary catheter from a patient not suffering from other "pathological conditions" to be negligence or malpractice because it would be causing death by omission. The law should look upon the provision of food and water in this way as well, and require its provision when withdrawal of successful food and water would result in death. Fr. O'Donnell's distinction is thus of value for these considerations, but it is a distinction that must be made with a great deal of care and precision.

Fr. O'Donnell's principles express classical Catholic medical ethical theory well, but it seems that they do not express sufficient consideration of the requirements of the common good. His criteria fail to give adequate consideration to the need of many competent and medically stable patients for greater protection than other patients and they place them in significant danger. His burden-benefit criteria are quite unclear and they could readily permit significant abuse and neglect of the medically stable incompetent by assertions that feeding could not provide to them.

Fr. O'Donnell's criteria are quite suitable for individual moral judgments, but it is not at all clear that they could provide an ethical foundation for adequate protection for medically stable patients or suicidal competent individuals.

## 5
### William E. May

Dr. William May has developed a comprehensive view of the nature of assisted feeding in an extended statement he authored and endorsed by a number of leading Catholic moralists. His statement is exceedingly important, and because it will have a profound effect on the Roman Catholic debate on this issue, and it can be found in the appendix of this chapter.

There seems to be some confusion in his theory as he generally seems to consider assisted feeding a medical treatment that should be provided according to the classical benefit-burden criteria, even though at the end of the statement he refers to it as elemental care that should be given even to the medically stable incompetent. May will not allow removal of food and water to cause death or because it is judged too burdensome. But one must ask how he can justify terming assisted feeding a "medical treatment" when he will not allow virtually any of the criteria traditionally employed to determine if "treatment" should be given to be used to govern these decisions.

He asserts that medical treatments are burdensome either in the strict sense when they are utterly pointless, or in the loose sense when their benefits are insignificant in comparison to their burdens. But it is hard to see how this loose sense could be applied to food and water when they can meet the nutritional and hydrational needs of the patient. If assisted feeding and fluids can be psychologically repugnant, the cause of great pain or physically damaging, they could be too burdensome.

May explicitly calls for laws to protect the medically vulnerable from deliberate killing by omission of required medical treatments, but one wonders if his theoretical account of the nature of assisted feeding and the conditions under which they have to be provided could do this. How the law could determine if a withdrawal or withholding of food and water was done to bring death or whether it was done to alleviate a burden that was unacceptable to the patient. If assisted feeding is considered an aspect of normal care, it would have to be administered except where death was truly imminent and its withdrawal would not be the fundamental and underlying cause of death, or where it could not be successfully administered. For if food and water can be removed to alleviate some severe burdens, and not to kill the patient, it would seem that those wanting to eliminate medically dependent patients would merely have to state that they did not intend the death of the patient, but only the removal of a burdensome or futile treatment. He says that one cannot remove feeding in order to kill a patient, but few euthanasiaists explicitly have that intention when they remove feeding. They argue for the removal of food and water to end suffering, be compassionate or show charity, and this rationale is not clearly addressed in his paper.

Because of this, it would seem that his principles can stand as an adequate ethical basis for the protection of medically vulnerable persons only with difficulty. This is important because courts might not always be able to distinguish different kinds of withdrawals caused by a choice against life from those caused by a choice for life. It is not clear that evidence could always be brought to a court to show that such a withdrawal was from an acceptable motive, and it would thus seem that this theory, consistent, comprehensive and persuasive as it is, could stand as the basis for such a law.

Nonetheless, May's analysis is excellent. The strength of his view is that it requires feeding for the medically stable, irrespective of their neurological condition. Professor May's theory could probably protect the incompetent person from being denied food and water, but it is not clear that his theory could require a competent person to receive them when failure to do so would be morally equivalent to suicide. It would seem that it would have been better for May to have argued that in those cases where the provision of assisted feeding by NG, IV or gastrostomy tube was medically possible, they should be considered as "normal care" and simply to be received by patients who are not imminently dying. Doing this would place the presumption in favor of feeding, and would make it more difficult to argue against their provision.

## 6
### Germain Grisez

Professor Germain Grisez has shifted his views on the issue of the nature of assisted food and water and on the conditions under which they must be provided. In *Life and Death With Liberty and Justice*, he held that normal care consisted of those things which patients would do for themselves if they were able, and it seemed that protection from exposure, sanitary care and the provision of nutrition and hydration were included in this category.[21] Later on, however, he revised this view and held that food and fluids were only medical treatments when they did not require the apparatus ordinarily used for medical care.[22] Grisez implied that normal care

---

[21] Grisez, Germain, and Boyle, Joseph. *Life and Death With Liberty and Justice*. (Notre Dame: University of Notre Dame Press, 1979.) P. 263.

[22] Grisez, Germain. "A Christian Ethics of Limiting Medical Treatment, Guidance For Patients, Proxy Decision Making, and Counselors." Lecture delivered at the Pope John Paul II Bioethics Center, Holy Apostles College and Seminary, Cromwell, Connecticut. Unpublished Manuscript. P. 7. *In the Matter of the Guardianship of Mary*

should simply be given to all patients, but this was not explicitly stated in his work.[23]

In an address delivered at the Pope John Paul II Institute for Bioethics, Grisez contended that food and water, when given intravenously or nasogastrically, are medical treatments, and he held that they should not have been given to Karen Quinlan after she left the hospital because she did not have a sufficiently strong claim to the resources required to provide them as she could not responsible to her social obligations.[24] Grisez's view was unique, because he was one of the few moralists considering this issue to hold that limitations on scarce resources could justify withholding or removing nutrition and fluids. He held that there was no duty to feed the persistently comatose, but this judgment would seem to be discriminatory because the comatose could derive the same benefits from feeding that others who are not neurologically impaired can receive from them.

Quite recently, however, Grisez changed his views, and he endorsed the statement authored by Dr. William May. Thus, he has reversed his views expressed in his address at the Pope John Paul II address and now endorses a very strict view of the conditions under which assisted feeding should be provided. In light the similarity of his views to those of Professor May, it is not necessary to specifically analyze his claims because what applies to Professor May's thought applies equally to Professor Grisez's.

## 7
### Edward Bayer

Fr. Edward Bayer has argued that nutrition when provided

---

*Heir*, 18 Mass. App. Ct. 200, at 201.

[23] Grisez, "A Christian Ethic", p. 8.

[24] Grisez, "A Christian Ethic", p. 8. Not even the President's Commission actually held that economic reasons could justify removal of food and water. However, Fr. John Paris has repeatedly mentioned cost considerations when speaking of the ethics of removing food and fluids from nonterminal comatose patients. He has not explicitly said that cost can justify their withdrawal, but he has considered it one factor which should be considered.

orally or "connaturally" should be considered as an ordinary means of sustaining life.[25] But when it is provided by assisted means it is "connatural" or a medical treatment that can become elective and extraordinary.[26] This distinction about the nature of the provision of assisted feeding is somewhat dubious and is not clearly helpful for supporting legislation because there are some times when the provision of assisted feeding is as mandatory as is oral feeding, and vice-versa. Is it more obligatory to provide spoon feeding to an Alzheimer's patient than it is to give a gastrostomy to someone such as Mary Heir? It would seem that in neither of these cases is feeding simply elective. Spoon feeding for an Alzheimer's patient has some of the characteristics of tube feeding and tube feeding for a patient like Mary Heir has some of the traits of oral feeding. Bayer's distinction that oral feeding is simply obligatory while assisted feeding is simply elective is too simple to deal with the complexities of caring for the disabled.

Bayer's theory could not stand as an ethical basis for a law protecting the medically vulnerable because his claim that the natural mode of feeding is obligatory and the "connatural" mode is elective would not impose any obligation whatsoever to give "connatural" feeding to the medically dependent. There are instances where assisted feeding is mandated by justice and it cannot simply be called elective just because it is not provided by assisted means. And there are some forms of assisted feeding that are required by justice and some forms of oral feeding that are elective. It is not the precise mode of delivery that makes feeding elective, but whether the withdrawal of feeding constitutes the fundamental and underlying proximate or remote cause of death that makes it mandatory or elective. Fr. Bayer so emphasizes the mode by which the patient receives food and water that he the obligation to give readily available life-sustaining food and water to the medically stable is obscured.

8

[25] Bayer, Edward. "Foregoing Life-Sustaining Food and Water: 1900 Years of Catholic Thought". Unpublished manuscript. P. 2.

[26] *Ibid.*

## Benedict Ashley, O.P.

Fr. Benedict Ashley understands the nature of assisted feeding and the conditions under which they should be given in much the same way that Fr. Kevin O'Rourke does. He argues that human bodily life shares in the dignity of the person, that it is always wrong to directly kill another person by either commission or omission, that appropriate technology must be employed by individuals to preserve their life and that this obligation is limited by the benefit and burden involved in the administration of care or treatment.[27] Fr. Ashley disagrees that assisted feeding is an aspect of normal care that should be given to all persons and he rejects claims that legislation should be promoted to require this for all patients.[28] He bases this position on the view that neither principle arguments for it are sustainable. Fr. Ashley asserts that the magisterium has authoritatively taught that assisted feeding is a medical treatment and that it is to be provided according to judgments of burden or benefit.[29] He notes that this is a papally confirmed judgment, and he argues that other documents must be understood in light of this one which leaves the question open.

He rejects the assertion that omitting assisted feeding is direct killing by the omission of obligatory care.[30] Only if it can be proven that the benefits of feeding outweigh the burdens of its provision is omission of feeding omission of appropriate care and that an obligation remained incumbent on the caregivers to provide

---

[27] Ashley, O.P., Benedict. "Financial Burdens and the Obligations to Sustain Life", Address to the Pope John XXIII Medical-Moral Research and Education Center Workshop for the U.S. Roman Catholic Bishops *Scarce Medical Resources and Justice*, February 9-13, 1987. Also see: "Hydration and Nutrition Consultation", a commentary on the paper *Feeding the Permanently Unconscious and other Vulnerable Adults*. Unpublished Manuscript. P. 1.

[28] "Hydration and Nutrition Consultation", P. 1.

[29] *Ibid*.

[30] *Ibid*. "The second was that to omit hydration and nutrition is to intend the death of the patient by omission of appropriate care. This would be true only if it could be proved that the benefit of such treatment to the patient always outweighed the burdens to the patient and to those who have the obligation to care."

the feeding. He asserts that feeding the comatose is not of benefit to them because there is no human way in which the feeding can be used by the person.[31] He claims that the use of assisted feeding for the comatose is intrinsically immoral because it is an application of technology that is disrespectful of human dignity.[32] And when this care places heavy psychological, economic and moral burdens on others, its use is immoral.

Fr. Ashley asserts that care could be removed when it imposed severe burdens on society or caregivers provided that society did what it could to prevent euthanasia.[33] But he proposes a looser understanding of the nature of benefit and burden. For him, considerations of burden and benefit should include not only considerations of the human bodily good, but also the total good of the human person.[34] This would seem to mean that if assisted feeding could sustain the life of the person, but could not support other bodily goods that it could or should be discontinued because it is useless or immoral.

He proposes that health care professionals should not be obliged to provide feeding to severely handicapped newborns or adults who cannot engage in conscious human acts.[35] He justifies

---

[31] *Ibid.*

[32] *Ibid.* "In the case of irreversibly comatose persons the artificial maintenance of human life which cannot be used in a human way may even be harmful, since it is an application of technology disrespectful of human dignity."

[33] *Ibid.* "I agree with those (Grisez, May, et al.) who held that such type (*sic*) of care can be omitted or discontinued when the benefits to life are outweighed by the burdens to the person or the care-takers or society, provided that in public policy and legislation we do what is possible to prevent abuse or the encouragement of euthanasia."

[34] *Ibid.* "But I would want to clarify this conclusion by insisting that while the benefit to the patient is the first consideration in any decision about care, the criteria for this "benefit" should be measured only in relation to the value of bodily life, but in terms of the total good of the human person in the hierarchy of human goods."

[35] *Ibid.* P. 2. "Consequently, it is not possible for those who care for irreversibly comatose persons or newborns so deficient as never to be able to engage in even minimally human acts to enable them to use their gift of life for the purpose for which God gave it, including the capacity to take food and fluids in a human manner. Therefore to prolong their life in an unconscious state by artificial means is not of

this by arguing that prolonging the lives of these individuals is of no benefit to them, and that bringing them to death should not be considered an unethical action. The only moral obligation incumbent on caregivers for these patients is to make them physically presentable to others and not offend the sensibilities of others in their treatment.[36] Doing this such that their "pathology" runs its course is the proper and appropriate course of treatment for them. Fr. Ashley objects that his arguments do not endorse dangerous "quality of life" arguments because he believes that those criticisms only apply when used to deny care and gradients to persons who are able to innocent individuals possessing normal quality of life.[37] He argues that "[s]uch arguments are dangerous only when they imply that it is permissible to directly intend the death of the innocent lacking a normal quality of life".[38] When a decision to not use assisted feeding stems from a judgment that it is not of benefit to a patient and that is a significant burden, that they are harmful or that they only prolong the dying process, it is not a proportionalist or "quality of life" judgment, but a legitimate assessment of the burdens and benefits of a medical treatment. He feels that "quality of life" only enters into the judgment because one

morally significant benefit to them. Since to do so for a long period is a serious burden to the care takers at least in the time, attention, and the psychological strain of awaiting death, it is not obligatory to undertake this burden for no significant benefit to the patient."

[36] *Ibid.* P. 2. "Therefore, the normal care for such patients is simply that required for the decent condition of the body in accordance with human dignity and the sensibility of others during the time that their pathology runs its inevitable course to death."

[37] *Ibid.* "But such arguments are dangerous only when they imply that it is permissible to directly intend the death of the innocent lacking a normal quality of life. The decision not to use artificial hydration or nutrition need not, however, stem from any intention of the death of the patient by omission, but first from the judgment that such procedures are of no significant benefit and are even harmful to the patient in that they prolong the inevitable dying process, and from the further judgment that such procedures involve disproportionate burdens to others at least because they involved prolonged care."

[38] *Ibid.*

must determine the degree to which care must be given to a patient.

Fr. Ashley is staunchly opposed to any legislation that would require feeding which a person might consider to be radically burdensome, but he does favor legislation that would protect comatose, incompetent or disabled persons from abuse or neglect.[39] He feels that legislation requiring feeding would actually promote euthanasia by making all opposition to it appear unreasonable and inconsistent.[40] The only legislation he would support would be that which would prevent abuses such as the denial of food and water to patients who are senile, brain damaged or incompetent to perform human acts.

However, one must ask how this sort of legislation could be consistently enacted because in American jurisprudence, rights to the competent readily become rights that are ascribed to the incompetent. Incompetency is not seen in American law as a condition which would deny a person the right to refuse treatment. If a competent person is allowed to reject feeding as being too burdensome, that right is going to be extended to the incompetent by surrogate, and there would be little way of protecting the incompetent from neglect and abuse.

Rather than protecting the medically vulnerable and incompetent from abuse and neglect, Fr. Ashley's criteria would seem to promote it. By arguing that the total human good must be promoted by assisted feeding, he is eliminating virtually all obligations to give feeding. By arguing that feeding is not only useless if a person has no capacity for conscious human acts, but that it is positively harmful to such persons, it would seem that Fr. Ashley is placing these permanently incompetent but nonterminal patients in serious jeopardy.

---

[39] *Ibid.* "Hence I would support only such legislation as would aim at preventing abuses such as the denial of hydration and nutrition to defective or senile or brain damaged persons who are still capable of a minimum of human conscious life."

[40] *Ibid.* "Consequently, I certainly would favor prudent legislation to outlaw euthanasia absolutely and to prevent neglect of comatose or senile or defective persons. But in framing and promoting such legislation we must take care not to impose as obligatory technical procedures which are seriously burdensome and which cannot be justified by the sound traditional practices of Catholic moral doctrine. To do so would in the long run promote the euthanasia movement by making all opposition to it appear unreasonable and inconsistent."

## 9
## Daniel Callahan

Daniel Callahan initially wrote that he was uneasy about removing food and fluids from patients because of the emotional significance of food and water.[41] But in a recently published article, he stepped back from his earlier view and held that food and water were merely medical treatments that could be provided according to standard medical criteria.[42] Callahan claimed that he could no longer consider these to be anything but medical treatments when administered under a physicians guidance. He believes that patients who succumb after a nasogastric tube or IV line are withdrawn do not die from the lack of basic resources of the body, but from the medical problem that caused the difficulty with swallowing.[43] This claim is somewhat opaque, however, when one considers that the symptoms associated with death by dehydration are usually more closely associated with that than with difficulties in swallowing.

His assertion that food and water have a special symbolic importance is not particularly helpful as there are many things and actions that have special symbolic importance but are not critical to us as is feeding. His understanding of the nature of feeding and medical treatment is so ambiguous as to be virtually of no help in understanding this issue. Callahan seems to not want to enter deeply into this discussion of the nature of assisted feeding to discover the nature of these treatments and to know when they are required or not. He does not tell us why food and water have "symbolic value" or why that value is so special that it should make us wary of withdrawing them.

There is simply very little in his thought that would in fact require their provision for patients. Affirming the symbolic value of food and water does not create any legal imperative to require their

---

[41] Callahan, Daniel. "On Feeding the Dying", *Hastings Center Report*, Vol. 131, No. 5, October, 1983. P. 22.

[42] Callahan, Daniel, "Feeding the Elderly Dying", *Generations*, Fall/Winter, 1986. P. 4.

[43] *Ibid.*

provision for patients. Callahan might have been better off saying that food and water are necessities of life that have to be given to patients, for if denied, the patient would certainly die. His assertion that food and water have symbolic value has an some "poetic" or "inspirational" value, but this tells us little of the moral requirements for their provision. Callahan's understanding of food and water seems to be a calculated study in ambiguity, for about all he is telling is us that they are important and we should be careful about dealing with them, but the precise and specific guidance we are searching for is lacking. Thus, his understanding is so cloudy as to make it an unsuitable ethical basis for protective legislation.

## 10
## William Smith

Msgr. William Smith has argued that the provision of assisted feeding and hydration is what he calls "minimal care", the bare minimum that must be provided to all patients by health care providers. He considers it to be a medical treatment, but a unique form of treatment, one that can become extraordinary in only the rarest of instances.[44] Smith is very strict in his requirements for providing nutrition and fluids, and he seems to allow it to be removed only when it is radically painful or when it cannot meet the nutritional and hydrational needs of the patient.[45]

Msgr. Smith has offered probably the best ethical account of the nature of food and water and criteria for their provision of any of the ethicists discussed. In holding that food and water are aspects of "minimal care" or medical treatment, he has placed them in the category of treatments whose withdrawal constitutes neglect

---

[44] Smith, Msgr. William. "Judeo-Christian Teaching on Euthanasia: Definitions, Distinctions and Decisions" *The Linacre Quarterly*, Vol. 54, No. 1, February 1987. P. 29.

[45] *Ibid.* Pp. 29-30. It is not quite clear under what conditions minimal care can be withheld or withdrawn, but it appears that these are the conditions which he espouses.

or deliberate killing by omission.[46] In doing this, he has done a great service as a serious problem in medical practice is that of determining if there are any forms of care that may not be omitted except in the most extreme and uncommon of circumstances. The majority of medical ethicists today argue against the existence of such a category of treatment, but Msgr. Smith has argued effectively that in behalf of such a category of treatment and that these forms of care that must be offered as a duty in justice. He denies that they are without benefit to a patient when they can meet the nutritional and hydrational needs of a patient, and he does not believe that arguments can be validly made that they are excessively burdensome for comatose patients. When they are withdrawn from medically stable patients, the patient is killed by their removal, and not merely "allowed to die".

What is ironic, however, about Msgr. Smith's position is that he does not believe that legislation should be enacted to require the provision of nutrition and fluids, as he believes that medical practice cannot be legally regulated and that attempts to regulate their provision would be open to constant legal revision by opponents.[47] While he has developed one of the best theories for the protection of the medically vulnerable, he is the most reluctant to allow their use for development of law to protect them because of its susceptibility to abuse and revision.

The report issued recently by the Pontifical Academy of Science for endorsement by Pope John Paul II held that nutrition and fluids had to be provided to all comatose patients, irrespective of their prognosis.[48] This was demanded by the Academy because nutrition and fluids were considered to be aspects of normal care and not medical treatments, and were to be provided whenever they

---

[46] *Ibid.* P. 29. For adult patients, he includes food, water, bed rest, room temperature and personal hygiene. For pediatric cases, he adds to these blood, oxygen and clearing air passages. He claims that what distinguishes these is that their removal is destructive and causes death.

[47] Personal Communication. April 17, 1987.

[48] Pontifical Academy of Sciences, "The Artificial Prolongation of Life and the Exact Determination of the Moment of Death", (October 30, 1987).

could sustain life.[49] This document is quite revolutionary because it has gone against the prevailing opinions of theologians to support the rights of the disabled and those on the edge of life which hold that nutrition and fluids when provided by intravenous line, nasogastric tube, hyperalimentation or gastrostomy are medical treatments and are to be administered according to the traditional criteria for providing medical treatments.

As a consequence of and in light of these views, I would like to argue in behalf of the principles enunciated in the report of the Pontifical Academy. To do this, I will first show that assisted nutrition and fluids are different from medical treatments, and that there should be different criteria governing their provision than should govern the provision of medical treatments. Then, I wish to assert that the understanding of the nature of assisted feeding that is most congruous with laws aiming at the protection of the medically vulnerable and the prevention of suicide is that which supports the views of the Pontifical Academy's report.

## B
## NUTRITION AND FLUIDS: ASPECTS OF NORMAL CARE

In a recent report issued by the Hastings Center, *Guidelines on the Termination of Life-Sustaining Treatment and the Care of the Dying*, it was explicitly affirmed that providing assisted feeding and fluids by nasogastric tube and intravenous line was an aspect of customary and ordinary care given to patients:

> All invasive procedures for supplying nutrition and hydration *all enteral and parenteral techniques* should be considered procedures that require the patient's or surrogate's consent, and procedures that the patient or surrogate may choose to forgo. This includes not only procedures such as use of a gastrostomy or jejunostomy tube, but also the nasogastric (NG) tube and the peripheral intravenous line (IV). The practice has been not to seek consent for these latter two procedures because they have

---

[49] *Ibid.*

been considered part of the routine care consented to on admission to the health care institution.[50][italics mine]

The *Herbert* court abolished the classical category of ordinary care and defined all procedures done to patients as medical treatments.[51] This court held it to be lawful to remove food and water from a nonterminal patient when there was only an uncertain neurological prognosis that the person would not regain neurological functioning.[52] The *Conroy* court held that an even less intrusive and risky means of providing food and fluids could be removed when there was only a vague judgment that the person would die within a year and when the person was in intolerable pain.[53] The *Conroy* court rejected the judgment of an appeals court which held that removing a nasogastric tube would be to inflict an independent lethal cause on the patient and is not the removal of a mere *causa prohibens*.[54] It also rejected the view that nasogastric feeding was an aspect of normal care that was to be given whenever and wherever it was medically possible to provide it.

The Clarence Herbert court tried to make the case that assisted feeding was comparable or identical to the provision of respirators. There are similarities between the provision of assisted feeding and respirators, for the denial of either oxygen or food and water makes death certain for both the healthy and the ill. But it is too simple to say that the two are simply comparable. Respirators impose a much greater burden on health care providers and the recipients than nasogastric feeding tubes. They require

---

[50] *Guidelines on the Termination of Life-Sustaining Treatment and Care for the Dying*, The Hastings Center, (Briarcliff Manor, New York: 1987) Part II, Sect. C, II, 9, B. P. 61

[51] Barber v. Superior Court, 195 Cal Rptr 484, (1983).

[52] See: Paris, J. "Court Responses to Withholding or Withdrawing Artificial Nutrition and Fluids", Pp. 2244-2245.

[53] *In re Conroy*, 446 A2d 303 *cert. granted*, 470 A2d 418 (1983).

[54] *Ibid.*

specialized medical and technical skills, while the skills required to provide nasogastric feeding are so minimal that laypersons can usually learn what is required in a matter of hours. Respirators impose much greater risks on patients than do nasogastric feeding tubes, and their failure is associated with medical emergencies more often than are failures of nasogastric tubes. Withdrawal of a respirator does not make death inevitable, while removal of a successful feeding tube makes death certain. The need for assisted feeding is not always and everywhere associated with a "lethal, fatal or certainly pathological condition" as it ordinarily is with the need for medical treatments.

Theologians such as Frs. Paris, McCormick, Ashley and O'Donnell and various courts such as the *Herbert*, *Conroy*, *Brophy* and *Jobes* courts argue that assisted feeding is either comparable to or identical with medical treatments and therefore should be applied in accord with the normal criteria employed to govern their provision. But food and fluids are not strictly comparable to medical treatments because they do not perform the same function in the body that medical treatments do. Nutrition and fluids have a finality and teleological orientation that is different from that of medical treatments, for they naturally meet the nutritional and hydrational needs of the body. This finality and teleological orientation distinguishes them from medical treatments which directly, proximately and immediately cure, remedy or palliate clinically diagnosable conditions. Medical treatments are *causae prohibens* which impede, remedy, cure or palliate previously existing clinical conditions. But nutrition and fluids have a different status. Definitive denial of nutrition and fluids imposes a new and independently existing lethal cause, while denial of medical treatments enables a previously existing pathological condition to progress without impediment. Food and fluids are employed universally by the body to sustain its natural functions and support its natural defenses against diseases. They are basic resources of the body and are of direct, immediate and proximate nutritional and hydrational value irrespective of the mode of their provision.

In some respects, assisted feeding can be compared to a mechanical respirator, but it can also be compared to a cane or walker, a tracheal tube and or long-wear contact lenses. Assisted feeding can be compared in some ways to a cane given a person who needs it for walking rather than to a respirator, as they both are simple devices which assist natural bodily functions. But an even greater similarity can be found between nasogastric feeding tubes and long wear contact lenses. These three are invasive and require some skill to create or implant, but when that is done usually only routine, customary, careful and skilled nursing care is required to be maintained. They all assist natural bodily functions and do not actively take over a bodily function as does a respirator.

The comparison between nasogastric feeding tubes and a tracheal tube is fitting, for just as one would give a tracheal tube to anyone who would be enabled to breath with it, so also one should give a nasogastric feeding tube to anyone whose life can be significantly sustained by its provision. The tubes themselves could conceivably be considered as a medical treatment because they are provided under the authority of a physician, even though they are inserted and maintained by nurses, but neither the air nor the food and fluids are medical treatments. (But if that were to be done, then walkers, tooth brushes and eyeglasses should also be considered medical treatments!) And withdrawing a tracheal tube when it can enable a person to successfully breathe should not be permitted, as this would cause death by suffocation. And tube feeding is different from the provision of such things as insulin for the reason that food is an extrinsic, natural resource of the body, while insulin substitutes for an intrinsically produced natural resource of the body.

Assisted feeding can also be compared to the provision of a urinary catheter. Unlike a respirator, nasogastric feeding tubes and catheters both operate within the same gastrointestinal and urinary systems. Both are passive devices, and just as one would not remove a successful urinary catheter from a patient, thereby causing the death of a patient who was medically stable with it, one should not remove successful feeding tubes from patients who was medically stable with assisted feeding.

There is a real difference, however, in the way that the removal of a respirator is associated with the death of the patient and the way in which removal of nutrition and fluids is associated with patient death. The lack of food and water *causes* death where no other pathological conditions prevail, while removal of a respirator often permits death to occur because of the failed respiratory function.[55] Withdrawing food and water is not an occasion but a cause of death because death can occur from its withdrawal in the absence of any other pathological condition. Death resulting from the removal of a respirator can only occur if there is a preexistent lethal cause.

The burdensomeness of assisted feeding does not make it a medical treatment, for they are often less intrusive or risky than walkers for the elderly, which are hard to consider as medical treatments. Nasogastric feeding tubes can be compared to walkers which supplement natural functions, even though they are not intrusive, and are not true medical treatments. Simply because NG tubes aid, but do not duplicate natural bodily functions, they are not simply medical treatments.

Morally speaking, definitively removing successful and readily providable food and water is different from the removal of a respirator because it is equivalent to an injection of poison because both make death certain for any individual irrespective of their clinical condition. Removing food and fluids is analogous to putting a plastic bag over someone's face because both cause certainly death by denying extrinsic natural resources of the body. Withdrawing readily available food and water by such means as spoon feeding, nasogastric feeding, IV feeding has the same effect as does or injecting them with poison: certain death. This effect is not realized when respirators are withdrawn, even when a person is brain dead, and this indicates a difference in these two forms of care and treatment. It is hard to imagine how the definitive and absolute removal of food and fluids just like air can ever improve the clinical picture of the patient. Respirators can be temporarily removed in the hope that so doing will improve the condition of the patient, but definitive denial of oxygen is certainly lethal, just as definitive denial of fluids and nutrition certainly brings death.

Classical medical standards and practice have considered food and water to be aspects of patient maintenance and normal care, but not medical treatments. There are certain functions of basic patient maintenance such as hygienic care, sleep and rest, exercise and protection from exposure that are not strictly speaking

---

[55] See: Smith, Msgr. William. "Judeo-Christian Teachings on Euthanasia: Definitions, Distinctions and Decisions", P. 29.

medical treatments. When these basic maintenance functions are neglected they can create pathological conditions which require the skills of a physician to cure, but prior to that point food and fluids remain aspects of patient maintenance.

## CONCLUSION

Dr. William May has argued that there should be legislation to achieve these goals, and while he asserts very strict standards for the provision of food and water, it is not clear that his understanding of assisted feeding as a medical treatment would do this support legislation that would do this. The view that nutrition and fluids are aspects of normal care and are not strictly equivalent to medical treatments seems to be most conducive to legislation that would prevent deliberate killing or suicide by omission of food and water in a way that the other standards could not fully guarantee. Affirming assisted feeding to be a medical treatment will not enable the law to prevent its removal from medically stable patients in a suicidal manner. Because patients are allowed to reject "medical treatments", the law could not prevent suicidal rejections of food and water if it were to be considered as a medical treatment. This, however, is not the only view that would do this, for considering food and water as "minimal care" as Msgr. Smith does, would do the same. The law has an obligation to prevent suicide and abuse of the medically vulnerable, and it cannot make subjective judgments about the burdens and benefits of care or treatment. The duty of the law is to assure that individuals are not denied benefits on the basis of unjust discrimination. If it sees that a form of care or treatment will bring the same benefits to one class of patients that it brings to others, it must guarantee that it is provided.

Regarding assisted feeding as a medical treatment that can be denied some classes of individuals for whom it provides the same benefit that it gives to others must be curtailed by courts. The only ethical understanding that can enable the court to consider assisted feeding in this way is that of regarding it as normal or minimal care because these understandings require its provision when its removal would the immediate, proximate and direct cause of death.

In accord with the Pontifical Academy of Science's statement, life-sustaining nutrition and fluids should be given to all comatose patients, and to all terminally ill patients whenever it is medically possible to do so. The governing principle should be that if the patient expires the cause of death should be the underlying pathological condition and not the lack of basic resources resulting from a freely made choice not to provide them. The only circumstances when there would not be a moral obligation to provide them is when it would not be medically possible to provide them and where their provision would not be expected to sustain life. Food and water are always of benefit to a patient when they sustain life, and they should be given whenever they can do this. They have a different finality from that of medical treatments, and because of that they should be provided according to principles that are different from those governing the provision of medical treatments. If a patient rejects food and fluids for medical reasons, there would seem to be no obligation to provide them, but if a patient rejects food and water for nonmedical reasons, they should be given.

# APPENDIX

# FEEDING THE PERMANENTLY UNCONSCIOUS AND OTHER VULNERABLE PERSONS

## Statement in Support of the New Jersey Catholic Conference

William E. May, Ph.D.
Department of Theology
Catholic University of America.
Washington, D.C.

Recent court cases (such as those involving Claire Conroy, Paul Brophy, and Nancy Ellen Jobes) have called attention to the moral and legal questions concerning the provision by tube of food and fluids to the permanently unconscious (e.g., those diagnosed as being in a "persistent vegetative state") and other serious debilitated by nondying persons. Is it ever morally right to withhold or withdraw such nutrition and hydration? If so, on what grounds? And what should be the role of the law?

Before answering these questions, we think it necessary to state several crucially important presuppositions and principles relevant to the subject and also to reject a rationale offered by some ethicists--and apparently accepted by most courts--for withholding and withdrawing food and fluids provided by tubes from the permanently unconscious and other seriously debilitated by nondying persons.

## Presumptions and Principles

1. Human bodily life is a great good. Such life is personal, not subpersonal. It is a good *of* the person, not merely *for* the person. Such life is inherently good, not merely instrumental to other goods.

2. It is never morally right deliberately to kill innocent human beings--that is, to adopt by choice and carry out a proposal to end their lives. (We here set aside questions about killing those who are not "innocent", i. e., those convicted of capital crimes, engages in unjust military actions, or otherwise attacking others.)

3. It is possible to kill innocent persons by acts of omission as well as by acts of commission. Whenever the withholding or withdrawal of food and fluids carries out a proposal, adopted by choice, to end the life, the omission of nutrition and hydration is an act of killing by omission.

4. The deliberate killing of the innocent, even if motivated by an anguished or merciful wish to terminate painful or burdened life--a deliberate killing that will henceforth be called "euthanasia"--is not morally justified by that motive.

4. Like other killing of the innocent, euthanasia can be carried out by acts of omission ("passive euthanasia") as well as by acts of commission ("active euthanasia"). This distinction makes no moral difference.

6. Euthanasia can be voluntary (of a person who gives informed consent to be killed), nonvoluntary (of a person incapable of giving informed consent), or involuntary (of a person capable of giving informed consent who does not give it).

7. For a person who consents to be killed, voluntary euthanasia is a method of suicide. Nonvoluntary and involuntary euthanasia violate not only the dignity of innocent human life by the right of the person who is killed not to be killed. The law of homicide should continue to apply to all forms and methods of euthanasia; none should be legalized. The law of homicide, in particular, must protect innocent human beings from being killed for reasons of mercy.

8. While competent persons have the moral and legal right to refuse any useless or excessively burdensome treatment. But great care must be exercised in reaching the judgment that a treatment is useless or excessively burdensome, they must exercise great care both in order to avoid any intention to end life on the grounds that it is devoid of intrinsic worth and in order to fulfill properly the responsibility to respect human life.

9. Likewise, those who have the moral duty to make decisions for noncompetent persons (such as infants or the permanently unconscious) have a moral right to refuse any useless or excessively burdensome treatment of them. This right must, however, be exercised with great care in order for avoid the temptation, unfortunately not uncommon in our society, of devaluing the lives of the noncompetent or regarding such persons chiefly in terms of the utilitarian values they may represent. Too often,

unfortunately, the judgment that a treatment is useless or excessively burdensome does not reflect serious consideration of the objectively discernible features of the treatment but is an expression of attitudes toward the life being created. Moreover, in order to protect the rights of the noncompetent and to promote the common good, sound public policy justified proper regulation by law of the scope of treatment decisions made by parents and other proxies (cf. the federal Child Abuse Amendments of 1984).

10. Human life can be burdened in many ways. No matter how burdened it may be, human life remains inherently a good of the person. Thus, remaining alive is never rightly regarded as a burden, and deliberately killing innocent human life is never rightly regarded as rendering a benefit.

## Contemporary Threats to the Dignity of Innocent Human Life

Some today morally approve and seek the legalization of euthanasia, both passive, voluntary and nonvoluntary. (At present, public advocacy of involuntary euthanasia is rare.)

One argument for euthanasia is based on the claim that competent persons have a right to be killed mercifully--"right to die"--when they think that they would be better off dead than alive.

Another argument for euthanasia is based on the claim that competent persons can refuse all treatment and may choose to do so precisely in order to end their own lives. Assuming or claiming that it is justifiable to refuse treatment on this basis, some proponents of euthanasia argue that ending life with another's help often would be quicker and easier than choosing death in this way.

Some proponents of euthanasia employ dehumanizing language to support their proposal that noncompetent persons should be killed when their lives are judged by others to be valueless or excessively burdensome. Those to be killed often are defined as nonpersons or are called "vegetables." Some in poor health but stable and non-terminal condition, who are not in imminent danger of death, are reclassified as "terminal". Others are defined as "brain dead". even though some spontaneous functioning of the brain persists and the strict clinical criteria for declaring brain death are not verified.

Certain people claim to oppose euthanasia and do not

advocate killing by acts of commissions, but nevertheless support the view that treatment may rightly be withheld from noncompetent, nonterminal persons simply because their lives are thought by others to be valueless or excessively burdensome. Adopting this rationale, and accepting the assumption that life itself can be useless or an excessive burden, some American ethicists, physicians and courts have judged that food and fluids may rightly be withheld or withdrawn from persons who are not terminally ill because they are permanently unconscious or otherwise seriously debilitated.

However, withholding or withdrawing food and fluids *on this rationale* is morally wrong, because it is euthanasia by omission. The withholding or withdrawing of food and fluids carries out a proposal, adopted by choice, to end someone's life because that life itself is judged by others to be valueless or excessively burdensome. Moreover, the withholding or withdrawing of food and fluids *on this rationale* should be interpreted to violate fundamental principles of American law and equity, since it explicitly sanctions status-based discrimination--i.e., discrimination based on the debilitated physical or mental condition of the person. Such discrimination becomes a new basis for deliberate killing by omission--killing that is not justified by the plain language of applicable statutory or constitutional law.

It is cause for very great alarm that some influential physicians, ethicists and courts have adopted this rationale for withholding or withdrawing food and fluids--and other means of preserving life--from some persons. For in adopting this rationale, they approve and legally sanction euthanasia by omission--deliberate killing--in some cases. In order to prevent the sanctioning, even unintended, of killing of the innocent, everyone with relevant competence, especially ethicists, religious leaders, lawyers, jurists, physicians and other health care personnel must repudiate the withholding or withdrawing of food and fluids on this rationale.

If it becomes entrenched practice to kill by omission certain sorts of persons whose condition is very poor and whose lives are judged by others no longer to be worth living, then this method of killing will surely be extended to many other persons. Most of the cases which have attracted attention thus far have involved the very severely brain damaged--those who are permanently unconscious, severely damaged by strokes, in advanced stages of dementia due to Alzheimer's or other disease, and so on. But various sorts of damage, defect, debility and handicap which burden human life occur in myriad degrees, so that there are always more and less severe cases differing from one another only by degree. Unfortunately, it is not, unfortunately, difficult to imagine a future America in which human life will be judged excessively burdensome for all persons who cannot care for themselves and have no one willing and able to care for them. Since dying of thirst and starvation can be often slow, very painful, and disfiguring, the demand will follow that death be hastened by legal overdoses or injections. Thus, ironically, the purportedly "dignified death" of those who die from dehydration and malnutrition would occasion demands for deliberate killing by commission because of the indignity involved in such a death.

### Use of Tubes to Provide Food and Hydration For The Permanently Unconscious And Others Seriously Ill Persons

Providing food and fluids to noncompetent individuals such as infants and the unconscious is, under ordinary circumstances, a grave duty. Deliberately to deny food and water to such innocent human beings in order to bring about their deaths is homicide, for it is the adoption by choice of a proposal to kill them by starvation and dehydration. Such killing can never be morally right and ought never to be legalized. It follows that it is never right and ought never to be legally permitted to withhold food and fluids from the permanently unconscious or from others who are seriously debilitated (e.g., with strokes, Alzheimer's disease, Lou Gehrig's disease, organic brain syndrome, or AIDS dementia) as a means of securing their deaths.

However, when specific objective conditions are met, the withholding and withdrawal of various forms of treatment, including the provision of food and fluids by artificial means, do not necessarily carry out a proposal to end life. One may rightly choose to withhold or withdraw a means of preserving life if the means employed is judged either useless or excessively burdensome. It is most necessary to note that the judgment made here is *not* that the person's *life* is useless or excessively burdensome; rather the judgment is that the *means used to preserve life* is useless or excessively burdensome.

Traditionally, treatments have been judged useless or relatively useless if the benefits they provide to a person are either utterly pointless (useless in the strict sense) or insignificant in comparison to the burdens the impose (useless in the wider sense). Traditionally, a treatment has been judged excessively burdensome whatever benefits it offers are not worth pursuing, for one or more of several reasons: It is too painful, too damaging to the patient's self and functioning, too psychologically repugnant to the patient, too restrictive of the patient's liberty and preferred activities, too suppressive of the patient's mental life, or too expensive.

If judging whether a treatment or a noncompetent person is excessively burdensome, one must be fair. If those making this judgment take into account the damaged or debilitated condition of the patient and so give greater weight to the burdens and less to the benefits than they would were the patient in better condition, they judge unfairly. The principle they assume can be used to rationalize discriminatory withholding or withdrawing of care from anyone whose condition is poorer than the standard set by some arbitrary norm for adequate quality of life.

An exhaustive examination of each of these factors is beyond the scope of this Statement. We stress, however, that considerable moral certainty is required to justify foregoing nutrition and hydration because error would result in inevitable death and where doubt exists one should always adopt the safer course in favor of continued life. For the same reason, if a rare circumstance in which nutrition or hydration may legitimately be foregone exists, then it should be identified with precision and care, and this would be especially necessary in the formulation of law and public policy.

Yet the damaged or debilitated condition of the patient has been the key factor taken into consideration in virtually all the recent court cases which have focused attention on the moral and legal questions concerning the provision of food and fluids to permanently unconscious or other severely debilitated but nondying individuals. Decisions have been made to withdraw food and fluids not because continuing to provide them would be in itself excessively burdensome but because sustaining life was judged to be no benefit to a person in such poor condition. These decisions have been unjust and, as noted above, they set a dangerous precedent for more extensive passive or even active euthanasia.

Nonetheless, *if it is really useless or excessively burdensome* to provide someone with nutrition and hydration, then these means may rightly be withheld or withdrawn, *provided* that this omission does not carry out a proposal to end the person's life, but rather is chosen to avoid the pointless effort or the excessive burden of continuing to provide the food and fluids.

Plainly, when a person is imminently dying, a time often comes when it is really useless or excessively burdensome to continue hydration and nutrition, whether by tube or otherwise. But the question that concerns us is not one about patients who are judged to be imminently dying but rather with persons who are not.

In our judgment feeding such patients and providing them with fluids by means of tubes is *not* useless in the strict sense because it does bring to these patients a great benefit, namely, the preservation of their lives and the prevention of their death through malnutrition and dehydration. We grant that provision of food and fluids by tubes or other means to such persons could become useless or futile if (a) the person in question is imminently dying, so that any effort to sustain life is futile, or (b) the person is no longer able to digest or use the nourishment thus provided. But unless these conditions are verified, it is unjust to claim that the provision of food and water is useless.

We recognize that the provision of food and fluids by IVs and nasogastric tubes can have side-effects (e.g., irritation of the nasal passages, sore throats, collapsing of the veins, etc.) that might become serious enough in particular cases to render their use excessively burdensome. But the experience of many physicians and suggests that these side-effects are often transitory and capable of being ameliorated. Moreover, use of gastric tubes does nor ordinarily cause the patient great discomfort. Initially, there may be gas pains and diarrhea, but ordinarily such discomforts are of passing nature and can be ameliorated. We thus judge that providing food and fluids to the permanently unconscious and other categories of seriously debilitated but nonterminal persons (e.g., those with strokes, Alzheimer's disease) does not ordinarily impose excessive burdens by reason of pain, damage to bodily self and functioning, psychological repugnance, restrictions on physical liberty and preferred activities, or harm to the person's mental life.

The question remains whether providing food and water in this way to these patients is excessively burdensome because of its cost. To answer this question, it is important to note, first, that the cost of providing food and water by tubal means is not, in itself, excessive. Such feeding is generally no more costly than other forms of ordinary nursing care (such as cleaning or spoonfeeding a patient) or ordinary maintenance care (such as maintenance of room temperature through heating or air conditioning), It must, however, be acknowledged that the care of nondying persons in very poor condition, some times over a long time, can be quite costly when taken as a whole. For instance, the care of anyone who cannot eat and drink in a normal way requires not only tubal nutrition and hydration, but a room, which must be supplied appropriately with heat and utilities, and regular nursing care to keep the patient clean, prevent bed sores and so on.

Some of these patients might be cared for at home rather than in an institution; the regular provision of food and fluids by tube is usually not too difficult or complicated to be done by people without professional training if they are properly instructed and supervised. This is not to say that care of such patients, when feasible, is not costly in time and energy. Like care for a baby, it must be carried on constantly; however such care is more difficult than care for a baby, since it is harder to care for an adult's large body than for a baby's small one.

But such care is not without its benefits. Since it is necessary to sustain life, such care benefits the nondying patient by serving this fundamental personal good--human life itself--which, as we have explained, remains good in itself no matter how burdened it becomes due to the patient's poor condition.

Moreover, caring for others expresses recognition of their personhood and responds appropriately to it. For example, care for a baby is the form parental love naturally takes; care for a helpless adult--family member, neighbor, or stranger,--expresses compassion and humane appreciation of his or her dignity. It also offers the possibility to the caregiver of nurturing such noble qualities as mercy and compassion.

It is possible to imagine situations in which a society might reasonably consider it too burdensome to continue burdensome to continue to care for its helpless members. For example, in some very harsh environments, natural disasters, and war situations, the more able can be forced to make hard choices between caring for themselves (and their children) and providing life-sustaining care for those who are gravely disabled and helpless. However, our society is by no means in such straitened circumstances--in the aftermath of nuclear destruction we may face such a situation, but we are surely not facing one now.

Some Americans might prefer to abandon to death those who require long term care at public or private expense. But comparing the costs of care with its benefits, only one who sets aside the Golden Rule will consider excessively burdensome the provision by our society of life-sustaining care to all its members who require it and can benefit from it. As the Catholic Church stated in its 1981 Document for the International Year of Disabled Persons: "The respect, the dedication, the time and means required for the care of handicapped persons, even of those whose mental faculties are gravely affected, is the price that a society should generously pay in order to remain truly human," To withhold or withdraw from those in poor condition the elemental care they need to survive would be to decide that our society no longer values its members insofar as they are persons with dignity--that is, with inherent value independent of what they can do and contribute--but only insofar as they are useful, or so long as their lives have sufficient quality.

We thus conclude that, in the ordinary circumstances of life in our society today, it is not morally right, nor ought it to be legally permissible, to withhold or withdraw food and hydration provided by artificial means to the permanently unconscious or other categories of seriously debilitated but nonterminal persons. Rather, food and fluids are universally needed for the preservation of life, and can generally be provided without the burdens and expense of more aggressive means of supporting life. Therefore, both morality and law should recognize a strong presumption in favor of their use. Furthermore, judgments that these means of supporting life have become optional in an individual case should be scrutinized with the utmost care to ensure that such judgments are not guided by a discriminatory attitude regarding the value of disabled persons' lives or by an intention of deliberately hastening the death of such persons.


Drafted by:

William E. May, Ph.D.

Rev. Robert Barry,O.P.
Germain Grisez, Ph.D.
Msgr. James McHugh, S.T.D.
Brian Johnstone, C.Ss.R.
Msgr. William Smith, S.T.D.
Gilbert Meilander, Ph.D.
Rev. John Connery, S.J., S.T.D.
Mark Siegler, M.D.
Msgr. Orville Griese, S.T.D.
Thomas Marzen, J.D.

# CHAPTER TEN
# LEGISLATING TO PROTECT MEDICALLY VULNERABLE ADULTS

## A
## JURISPRUDENTIAL PRINCIPLES FOR THE CARE AND TREATMENT OF MEDICALLY VULNERABLE PERSONS

Because of the advent of the euthanasia movement, medically vulnerable persons could be deliberately killed by others, not only by denial of food and fluids, but also by denial of clinically beneficial medical treatments and care or by calculated benign neglect. The following are jurisprudential principles for protecting medically vulnerable persons from deliberate abuse and neglect, derived from the Nursing Home Action Group's guidelines for supportive care, are here set forth as moral guidelines for the development of protective legislation for medically vulnerable persons.[1]

1. *The life of the person with a mental or physical disability has the same intrinsic value as that of a person considered to be normal or able-bodied.*

2. The primary aim of caregivers is to promote and support the highest physical, mental, spiritual, emotional, and social life possible for the medically vulnerable person.[2]

3. Denial of beneficial, life-sustaining medical treatments and

---

[1] The aim of providing medical care and treatment is to promote and protect human life. In what promises to be a very influential book, Leon Kass, M.D,. has argued that the promotion of health is the primary aim of medicine. This view is inadequate for two reasons. First, in practice, physicians aim at protecting and promoting life, and they are not betraying their professional goals for so doing. Physicians object to participating in the execution of criminals not just because such participation involves them in the destruction of health, but in the destruction of life. Physicians aid the starving in Ethiopia who are on the brink of death, knowing that they will not able to restore full health, but they continue their efforts because they seek to preserve life.

The second reason why this principle is objectionable is that it implicitly admits that life need not be protected when health cannot be preserved. The fact that Kass refuses to explicitly condemn killing the imminently dying who are in serious pain suggests that he recognizes that his perspective tacitly allows mercy killing by positive measures or benign neglect. See: *Toward a More Natural Science*, (New York: Basic Books) 1986, p. 201.

[2] Any law asserting this requirement to report suspected cases of medical neglect or abuse should have the added requirement that no individuals who report such cases can be released from their position of employment within a specified period of time after reporting these cases unless there is clear and documented evidence of negligence.

normal care is a violation of the moral rights of the medically vulnerable person, and these courses of action should never be suggested to them. The law should require that anyone having knowledge of or suspecting denial of beneficial medical treatments or normal care from a medically vulnerable person to report this to law enforcement authorities.[3]

4. No medically vulnerable person should be forced to choose between length of life and quality of life. Considerations of economic policy should not be used to deny elderly, handicapped, poor, infirm, or disabled persons routine, customary and normal care.[4] Routine and customary care should be understood as protection from exposure, sanitary care, psychological support, and life sustaining food and water that can be provided under the conditions outlined in section IV, part 2.

5. The best interests of the medically vulnerable person are paramount. Preserving, extending, enhancing and making more comfortable the life of the medically vulnerable person are always in the best interest of the person, regardless of physical or mental condition.

---

[3] The only justification for refusing to offer those who suffer from handicap, chronic illness or disability routine, customary, and normal care is a quality of life judgment. But such an attempt to justify withholding these is inadequate because it would necessarily hold that persons with these debilities and handicaps do not have lives that are worth the expense of treatments. This type of justification requires that one make an assessment of the value of another's life, which is impossible to do objectively and in accord with justice. This form of justification is also erroneous for the reason that normal, routine and customary, care is not radically burdensome financially. Extraordinary medical treatments, such as bypass surgery or organ transplants can be extremely costly and of limited clinical benefit to patients, but these medical treatments are of a completely different order from patient maintenance, routine and customary care.

[4] When patients refuse to consent to beneficial medical treatments and routine customary care, there should be a presumption of incompetence. But when they request these, the presumption should be in favor of their competence. What was particularly outrageous about the Ella Bathhurst case was that there was no evidence whatsoever that she was consulted about her medical care. Physicians claimed that she suffered from "chronic brain syndrome" which is an extremely vague category of neurological deterioration. What was ignored by these physicians, however, was that the nursing staff repeatedly noted that she was hard of hearing. A speech pathologist was able to bring her to swallow by giving her clear and patient instructions to swallow food and fluids given her. See: Investigative Report # V85-299, Department of Health, State of Minnesota, July 12, 1985, and NRL News, September 26, 1985, 12, 16. pp. 1, 11.

6. The legally and clearly competent medically vulnerable person should be encouraged to participate in decision-making to the fullest extent possible.[5]

7. Decisions about medically vulnerable persons who are:
   a. severely disabled in any way;
   b. poor;
   c. leaving an inheritance; or
   d. without close friends or relatives should be monitored with particularly close attention.

8. Medical and nursing staff should not assist in suicide. Anyone who knowingly and willfully aids, abets, assists, advises, or encourages another to commit suicide, or who knowingly and willfully provides to, delivers to, or procures for another any drug or instrument knowing that the other may attempt to commit suicide with the drug or instrument shall be guilty of the crime of assisted suicide.[6]

---

[5] Only a minority of states have laws explicitly prohibiting assisted suicide. See D. Humphry, *Let Me Die Before I Wake*, 1984, at 97-99. In Texas last year, murder charges were withdrawn in the case of Air Force S/Sgt Joseph Dixon who placed all of the food in house out of the reach of his elderly mother who starved to death as a result because there were no explicit statutes requiring children to feed their parents. See: *Newsweek*, September 23, 1985, p. 42.

The Dixon case and the case of Betty Rollin suggest that suicide laws need to be strengthened. Rollin reported in her best selling book *Last Wish* how she and her husband helped Ida Rollin kill herself. If the accounts in the book are true, then Ms. Rollin's husband should be prosecuted for assisted suicide because he procured drugs which he knew Ida Rollin was going to use for her suicide. See: *Last Wish*, (New York: Simon & Schuster, 1985, pp. 190-1, 194. It is imperative that those who assist in the suicides of others be prosecuted so that contempt for the law against suicide is not allowed to grow.

[6] This stipulation would call many living wills into question because they are so vague and general. Living wills generally give competent patients the power to direct some aspects of their medical treatment. But they cannot cover every possible instance, and thus they are not helpful in determining what the patient's wishes are concerning a particular treatment. Also, very few of these advanced directives enable a patient to call for administration of normal care and ordinary medical treatments, and thus they are biased in favor of nontreatment. For an example of the ambiguity in some living wills, see: Society for the Right to Die. *Handbook of Enacted Laws*, (New York: Society for the Right to Die, 1985) p. 42. Describing the Nevada Living Will Act, it points out that a terminal condition is defined as any incurable condition "which is such that the application of life-sustaining procedures serves only to postpone the moment of death." This understanding of a terminal condition would include diabetes and it is highly likely that

# CONCLUSION

9. Greater protection must be afforded to the lives of medically vulnerable persons who refuse medical treatments. Before a facility or medical professional complies with a refusal-of-treatment request, it should be clearly documented in the medical records that:
    a. the medically vulnerable person was clearly competent;
    b. the medically vulnerable person made the request freely and without duress;
    c. the medically vulnerable person's intentions were clearly and accurately interpreted;[7]
    d. it has been determined by clinical evaluation that the medically vulnerable person was not suffering from psychological depression or the effects of chemical use;[8]

---

it would require that insulin be removed from a healthy middle aged male who had a nervous breakdown. It is not at all clear that many competent patients would consent to such a treatment policy.

[7] This is an exceedingly important stipulation. A recent study showed that the *vast* majority of terminally ill persons did not want to die, and those who did were notable for their advanced clinical depression. See: "Terminally Ill in Study Shun Euthanasia", St. Paul Pioneer Press and Dispatch, February 9, 1986, p. 17A. This study, conducted by Dr. James Henderson Brown of the University of Manitoba found that of 44 patients, only those who suffered from severe depression expressed a desire to receive mercy killing. Dr. Brown asserted: "It would appear that patients with terminal illness who are not mentally ill are no more likely than the general population to wish for premature death." This finding suggests that euthanasia is most attractive to those who are most vulnerable: those who are clinically depressed, despairing and mentally ill.

In one of the more famous cases concerning mercy killing, Elizabeth Bouvia asked that she not be given feeding by any form, but only painkillers so that she could painlessly die with dignity and thus be freed from her "useless" body. There is good reason to believe, however, that she suffered from deep depression. Married in August 1982, her husband left her a year later, and she has recently been connected to a morphine pump which regularly administers morphine injections upon demand. See: *Elizabeth Bouvia v. County of Riverside*, Cal. Super. County of Riverside. Slip opinion. No 159780, February 4, 1984.

Similarly, Ella Bathhurst is reported to have said that she wanted to die, but nurses repeatedly noted that she was severely depressed. This statement was used by physicians to justify withdrawing all fluids from her, yet none of these physicians intervened to either provide or call for psychological or psychiatric assistance for her. See: *Investigative Report* #V85-299, Minnesota Department of Health, p. 2, 4.

[8] In the Ella Bathhurst case, for example, the physicians did not even attempt to gain permission to implant a NG tube because they felt that Mrs. Bathhurst's daughter would never grant permission for it, which seems to have been a violation of this principle. See *Investigative Report*. #V85-299, Minnesota Department of Health, p. 16. This is a

e. the medically vulnerable person was fully informed of the available treatments along with other options and the consequences of noncombatant;[9]

f. the medically vulnerable person was encouraged to and given time to reconsider the decision;

g. possible extenuating environmental factors were considered as potentially influencing the decision of the medically vulnerable person;[10]

h. the medically vulnerable person was given the opportunity to summon family members, friends, advocates, and professionals to consider alternatives to the rejection of treatments.[11]

standard requirement of the medical principle of informed consent, but the Bathhurst case shows that it is probably violated quite frequently in the breach. One wonders how well respected it would be with patients who had signed living wills. Studies are needed to see if those who have signed such directives actually have made fully informed decisions to reject or receive specific medical treatments.

[9] As far as possible, medical professionals should attempt to determine if discriminatory social, familial or economic factors have entered into decisions by surrogates to withhold or withdraw beneficial care and treatments, for these persons should be protected from such judgments. Whenever possible, those responsible for the care of medically vulnerable adults should be free to challenge decisions to withhold or withdraw care on the suspicion that they might be based on discriminatory motives or an intention to bring harm to the medically vulnerable person. Under no circumstance should medical professionals permit decisions based on the view that the life of the medically vulnerable person has become a burden and that continued existence constitutes in and of itself a harm to the person to determine the level of care or treatment provided.

[10] Part of ordinary nursing routines requires nurses to consult with patients to determine who their friends or advocates are who could discuss treatment decisions with them. Doing this would give medically vulnerable persons time to assess their condition, prospects and abilities to cope with their condition. The institution's human rights committee should not permit withdrawal of care and treatment unless it has been certified that the patient has had an opportunity to consult with his or her friends, family, and advocates. See: Hoyt, Jane, D; and Davies, James. "A Response to the Task Force on Supportive Care", *Law Medicine and Health Care*, Vol. 12, No. 3, p. 104.

[11] This was not done in the Bathhurst case, and apparently there was no attempt made to assure that she understood the decision. In fact, it seems that everything possible was done to conceal the nature of the decision from her. See: *Investigative Report* #V85-299, Minnesota Department of Health. Failures to provide full documentation should be reported to proper authorities as suspected cases of medical abuse. This is

## CONCLUSION

10. When a major medical or life-and-death decision involves a questionably competent adult, a friend, family member, or advocate sincerely and demonstrably interested in promoting the life and wellbeing of the medically vulnerable person should assume responsibility of guardianship.

11. If a decision to limit treatment for a medically vulnerable person has been made, it should be fully documented that the guardian fully understood the decision and its consequences.[12]

12. Emergency medical treatment should be given to any medically vulnerable person in the event of injury or accident.

13. Terminally ill persons, as all other persons, should be given emergency treatment for accident or injury not related to their terminal illness.

14. When it becomes clear that a person is irreversibly, irreparably and terminally ill and that death is unavoidable and immediately present, food, fluids and medical treatments may be withdrawn, but whatever physical comfort that can be given the medically vulnerable person should be given.[13]

   a. As with all other medical care, this decision should be open to periodic evaluation.

   b. All medical and nursing treatments and care necessary for comfort should be provided.

15. A medical plan including a "death-allowing-care-goal" should be reviewed weekly by the attending physician and renewed if still

---

needed because a large majority of death certificates do not reveal the true nature of death, according to many studies, as was true with the Ella Bathhurst case. Fully documenting decisions to withdraw treatment is often the only way of verifying well concealed cases of medical abuse, neglect or mercy killing. Had there been fuller documentation of the condition of Clarence Herbert after his surgery, it is likely that disputes would not have broken out as these would have clarified questions about his true medical condition.

[12] Remarkable about the Ella Bathhurst, the Crista Nursing Home, and the currently pending August Hills nursing home cases is that painkillers were apparently not provided to any of these patients who died from either neglect,, starvation or dehydration. See: "Nursing Home Told to Prepare Guidelines on Life-Support", *The Seattle Times*, May 6, 1985, pp. 1, 11.

[13] See: J. Hoyt and J. Davies, "A Response to the Task Force on Supportive Care", *Law, Med. & Health Care*, 13, 3, p. 104, col. 1.

appropriate.[14] A "death-allowing-care-goal" is a decision to permit a known and certainly lethal cause to run its course unimpeded. This differs from a decision to kill by euthanasia or benign neglect because it does not introduce a new and independent lethal cause, but only allows a previously existing cause to proceed without impediment.

    a. If this care goal is renewed twice, or if it is questioned for any reason whatsoever, an independent second opinion must be obtained.[15]

    b. It will be the responsibility of the primary physician to provide written notice to all parties involved in the decision that this type of decision may hasten death.[16]

16. Medical orders and nursing care must reflect the needs of each individual medically vulnerable patient.

17. When doubts about the prognosis of a medically vulnerable person cannot be resolved, full curative treatments should be provided.

18. If a decision is made to provide only comfort care for a

---

[14] The aim of this second opinion would be to see if the patient's condition was in fact irretrievable. If such a care goal had to be renewed twice, it is highly likely that the person is not imminently dying and that beneficial medical treatments and normal care would be of benefit to the patient.

[15] Explicitly stating the probable results of withdrawal of even minimal care should be required to make those responsible for treatment decisions both fully aware of and fully responsible for their decisions. In the Clarence Herbert case, it was not completely evident to Mrs. Herbert that removing her husband's respirator and fluids line would in fact hasten his death. If it was clearly stated that withdrawal of these devices would hasten his death, consent for their removal might not have been given so readily. See: Horan and Grant, *Legal Aspects*, *supra*, note 31, p. 604.

[16] This requirement is necessary for the reason that some residential facilities apparently reduce all care when comfort care alone is given. This is what apparently happened at the August Hills home where a number of elderly persons were brought to death by severe neglect. 87-year-old Eleanor Breed died of starvation worsened by bedsores and spreading infections in 1978. Edna Mae Witt died 45 days after admission after she developed twenty-one bedsores including a 2-by-3 inch bedsore that was more than an inch deep which resulted in septicemia. See: "Murder Trial Resumes as Nursing Home Presents Its Defense", *American Medical News*, January 17, 1986, p. 5. This requirement is also needed for patients with chronic illnesses or handicaps, who need minimal nursing care and routine treatment. To lower care for patients with these conditions would be to cause their deaths.

patient, the standards of medical and nursing care must *not* be lessened.[17]

19. Environmental factors must be considered whenever "Supportive-Care-Only" orders are given. These orders require that only nutrition, fluids, hygienic care, protection from exposure, and psychological support, but no curative or remedial medical treatments be given to a patient.

The following factors, which may influence the issuing of such orders must be considered:

    a. the social services and medical and nursing care of the facility;

    b. the capacity of the environment to encourage meaningful, supportive interaction between the medically vulnerable persons and others;

    c. the provision of life-enriching activities and encouragement to participate in such activities; and

    d. whether the medically vulnerable person is free from medications which may cause loss of motivation, diminished activity, or other side-effects.[18]

20. If a medically vulnerable person has made a decision concerning care and treatment in advance, medical and nursing personnel must be alert to changes of mind by the person after execution of his or her previous decision.

21. If there is any reasonable evidence that a medically vulnerable person has had a change of outlook on life after a

---

[17] Psychoactive drugs can often have a bearing on the desire of patients to receive care and treatment, not to mention their desire to be treated. This seems to have been what happened to Elizabeth Bouvia to an extreme degree, and it probably happens to other patients to a much lesser degree. Writing "Supportive-Care-Only" guidelines for those under the influence of these medications presents the risk of violating the right of patients to fully informed consent as patients must be free from medically induced limitations on their freedom and abilities to cope with reality. See: Hoyt & Davies, "A Response to The Task Force on Supportive Care", p. 103-5, 134.

[18] This stipulation is needed because of the Crista Nursing Home incident where six nurses were threatened with demotion or transfer to other positions because they objected in conscience to removing a feeding tube from patients whom they judged to be responsive and medically stable. "Conscience clauses" are needed as much for health care staff in withdrawal of treatment cases as in abortion cases. "Wrongful Firing Charged in Euthanasia Case", *The Seattle Times*, October 10, 1985, p. C4.

decision to refuse care or treatment, this shall take precedence over any prior decision.

22. It is the responsibility of the health care facility to remind residents and guardians that independent advocates such as ombudsman programs or legal services programs are available, and to assist medically vulnerable persons in contacting these individuals or organizations.

23. Nurses or other health care professionals should not be subjected to demotion or release for refusing to comply with orders to downgrade or deny what they judge to be beneficial care or treatment.[19]

24. Within each health care facility, a human rights committee should be established to advocate the rights and quality of services due all residents. The committee would function independently of the staff and would be staffed by family and friends of the residents, rehabilitation personnel from outside the facility, community members, and religious leaders.[20]

## B
## PROTECTING MEDICALLY VULNERABLE ADULTS
## 1
## THE FEDERAL ROLE

The emergence of the mercy killing movement in this country will not only increase the number of voluntary suicides, but the emergence of nonvoluntary mercy killing will place people of questionable maturity and competence in jeopardy. As the AIDS

---

[19] Such a human rights commission would have the explicit function of promoting the reception of ordinary and beneficial medical treatments and routine and customary medical treatments. It would also have the aim of assuring that the highest quality of medical services is promoted. Measures to assure that there are no conflicts of interest between the committee, the health care institution, and insurers should be taken. Review of the proceedings of such committees should be periodic. Committees should be bound by the moral obligations that should govern infant care review committees. Enactment of legislative measures based on these to protect medically vulnerable adults would seem to be in accord with the principles enunciated in the Older Americans Act. See: *Older Americans Act* of 1965, 42 U.S.C. 3001 (1982).

[20] Sacred Congregation for the Doctrine of the Faith, *Declaration on Euthanasia*, 1981, Sect. 4.

crisis deepens, it is quite probable that more and more medically vulnerable and dependent people will either willfully end their lives and that more medically vulnerable persons will be involuntarily end their lives.

This is seen most clearly in a recent report that one out of every eight patients who died in Holland from AIDS died from a physician administered lethal injection.[21] It is also seen in the fact that the Dutch Health Council is considering an amendment to proposed euthanasia legislation that would permit terminally ill minors to receive lethal injection without the consent of their parents. In the first case, AIDS patients, who are medically vulnerable adults are being denied medically beneficial treatments, and in these incompetent minors are denied the protections of their guardians or parents, which violates their rights to full protection from abuse and neglect.

That the mercy killing movement will violate the rights of the medically vulnerable to minimal and basic care is seen by the Bathhurst, Brophy and Jobes cases. Where it was never fully clear that they sought to be deliberately starved or dehydrated to death. In order to prevent medically vulnerable and incompetent patients from being exploited by the emergence of the mercy killing movement I will suggest in this chapter that various legal remedies be sought to enhance protections for these classes of patients.

It is of utmost importance is for the federal government to see its role in protecting the medically vulnerable and incompetent. One might ask why the federal government should become involved in this in light of the fact that mercy killing involves violations of the law on homicide, which has traditionally been reserved to the states. The crucial point is that mercy killing involves breaches of the civil rights of the disabled, incompetent and medically vulnerable by denying them forms of treatment and care from which they could readily and clearly benefit. Mercy killing, and particularly mercy killing by omission of readily available beneficial medical treatments and denial of readily available and beneficial nutrition and fluids involves denying these patients a benefit that is accorded to other classes of citizens, but denied them.

While the federal government cannot enforce laws against

[21] CBS Radio News, April 1, 1987

homicide or suicide, it can justifiably require the states to abide by equal protection laws. For example, section 504 of the Rehabilitation Act prohibits denial of beneficial medical treatments to infants based on their disability, which it construes to mean mental or physical disability, and this law should be applied equally to medically vulnerable adults. If this would not be successful, then similar measures could be enacted under the Older Americans Act. Decisions made by families or health care providers to withhold or withdraw beneficial medical treatments or food and water are not simply and solely medical decisions, but are decisions that also have a discriminatory character to them. For these individuals would not deny food and water to patients without their prognosis or diagnosis if the food and water was of benefit to them.

Could federal law require that medical treatments and food and water be given to patients who do not consent to receive it? It would seem that there would be some grounds for saying that it could. For federal law can prohibit individuals from entering into relationships detrimental to their well being with their consent. The jurisprudential basis that law has is the interest of the law in preventing suicide.

If the law were to give unrestricted permission to individuals to reject whatever beneficial medical treatments they chose or to reject food and water when these could be readily provided, sustain life meaningfully and not cause undue pain, it would implicitly undermine the law on suicide and allow many vulnerable persons to be exploited by others Permitting suicide would place the immature and mentally disabled in severe jeopardy because they are most at risk of ending their own lives and make them more vulnerable to exploitation by others. In order to protect these extremely vulnerable and fragile people from themselves, federal law could significantly restrict the rights of others in order to protect these people from exploitation and abuse. If the mentally and immature were not in serious danger of self inflicted death, it might speculatively be possible to give wide-ranging freedom to others to reject beneficial medical treatments in a wide variety of circumstances. But because the laws has an obligation injustice to be biased in favor of protecting the fragile rights and lives of the weak, poor and vulnerable, it is justified in placing restrictions on some of the rights of others.

We thus see that the federal government does have a significant role in protecting the lives and rights of the vulnerable from the mercy killing movement. In the following section, I wish to outline in detail what the role of the states must be in protecting medically vulnerable adults.

## 2
## THE ROLE OF THE STATES:
## MODEL LEGISLATION FOR THE PROTECTION OF MEDICALLY VULNERABLE ADULTS

In order to properly protect the medically vulnerable from medical neglect and abuse, it would be of value to enact at the present time legislation that offers them sufficient protection. In what follows, I wish to suggest three model statutes to protect them.[22]

### PREVENTION OF ASSISTED SUICIDES ACT

*Suggested Legislation*

(Title, enacting clause, etc.)

Section 1. [*Short title.*] This act may be cited as the *Prevention of Assisted Suicides Act*. [An amendment to the state criminal code]

2. [*Suicide -- Unlawful Suicide -- Unlawful Act.*] A person shall be guilty of a [serious felony] who intentionally, knowingly, or willfully:
(A) Aids, abets, assists, advises, or encourages another to commit suicide, or who
(B) Provides to, delivers to, or procures for another any drug or instrument with knowledge that the other may attempt to commit suicide with the drug or instrument.

---

[22] Thanks must be given to David Shaneyfelt of the National Legal Services Corporation, Joseph Piccione of the National Forum Foundation for their assistance in the development of these model statutes.

Section 3. [*Failure to Commit Not a Defense.*] Failure of another to commit suicide shall not be a defense to a person charged with committing an act under Section 2.

Section 4. [*Severability clause.*]

Section 5. [*Repealer clause.*]

Section 6. [*Effective date.*]

(Add as an amendment to the wrongful death statute of the state civil code):

"Any person who aids and abets the suicide of another may be civilly liable for the wrongful death of the suicide victim."

# THE BASIC NURSING CARE AFFIRMATION ACT

Suggested Title

(Title, enacting clause, etc.)

Section 1. [*Short title.*] This act may be cited as the Basic Nursing Care Affirmation Act.

Section 2. [*Purpose.*] The legislature hereby recognizes the cherished role of medical caregivers in our society, and the importance of preserving high standards of care. In recognizing the difference between treatment and care, it is the purpose of this Act to:

(A) Ensure traditional medical and nursing practices for providing care;

(B) Establish that all patients are entitled to ordinary and basic care, without regard to whether they are competent to participate in decisions regarding care;

(C) That nutrition and hydration are components to the care to which all patients are entitled; and

(D) That failure to provide proper care is a breach of medical ethics and subject to penal sanction.

Section 3. [*Construction.*] This act shall not be construed to supercede any authority or actions to be taken by other appropriate law-enforcement authorities, or to limit any cause of action applicable at common law or by other statute. This Act shall be liberally construed to effect its purpose.

Section 4. [*Definitions.*]

(A) "Attending physician" means the physician with primary responsibility for the care and treatment of a patient. If there is more than one physician caring for the patient, these physicians among themselves, shall designate the "attending physician" for purposes of this Act.

(B) "Facility" means a hospital or other entity required to be licensed pursuant to [appropriate chapter relating to hospitals and medical facilities]; a nursing home required to be licensed to serve adults pursuant to [appropriate chapter relating to nursing homes]; an agency, day care facility, or residential facility required to be licensed to serve adults pursuant to [appropriate chapter]; or a home health agency certified for participation in Titles XVIII or XIX of the Social Security Act, United States Code, title 42, secs. 1395 et seq.

(C) "Life-sustaining procedure" means any medical procedure or intervention that uses mechanical or other artificial means to sustain, or supplant a vital function of a person terminally ill and serves only to artificially prolong the moment of death. "Life-sustaining procedure" does not include the usual care provided to patients, which would include routine care necessary to sustain patient comfort and the usual and typical provision of nutrition which in the medical judgment of the attending physician such person can tolerate, and subject to the provisions of Section 6.

(D) "Patient" means any natural person admitted to a facility.

(E) "Physician" means an individual licensed to practice medicine by the [appropriate state board of medical examiners].

(F) "Terminally ill" means the incurable condition of a person caused by injury, disease or illness, which regardless of the application of life-sustaining procedures will, within reasonable medical judgment, produce imminently and where the application of life-sustaining procedures serve only to postpone the moment of death of the person.

Section 5. [*Basic Care Mandated*.] A Facility shall provide each patient with all elements of basic care: necessary food, water, clothing, shelter, hygienic care, and skilled nursing assistance.

Section 6. [*Necessary Food and Water*.] For purposes of Section 5, necessary food and water means nutrition and hydration, irrespective of the manner of provision or assistance, sufficient to maintain the patient at his highest possible level of heath as determined by his attending physician in accordance with ordinary and accepted standards of medical care, but does not include nutrition and hydration, when, in the judgment of the patient's attending physician and a second consulting physician:

(A) The administration of nutrition and hydration will, in an of itself, cause severe, intractable, unavoidable and long lasting pain to the patient.

the patient.

(B) The administration of nutrition and hydration is not medically feasible, in that:
>    1. The patient is unable to ingest nutrients or incorporate fluids, or
>    2. No technique or procedure reasonably available to the attending physician for such administration; or

(C) The death of the patient cannot be avoided, even by the provision of nutrition and fluids.

Section 7. [*Discrimination Prevention.*]

(A) No person may be forced to waive the elements of care in Section 5 as a prerequisite to admission to a facility, or to coverage under a policy of insurance of health care plan.

(B) The durable power of attorney, as provided in [appropriate section relating to durable powers of attorney], shall not be construed to make on behalf of a patient a directive to forego life-sustaining or life-resuscitating procedures.

(C) The law of this State shall not be construed to warrant discrimination based solely on the mental status or disability of a patient in the providing of medical treatment or care.

Section 8. [*Penalties.*] Any facility which intentionally, knowingly or willfully fails to provide necessary food and water to a patient under its care shall be guilty of a [misdemeanor].

Section 9. [

*Severability clause.*]

Section 10. [*Effective date*]

## THE MEDICALLY VULNERABLE ADULTS PROTECTION ACT

## SUGGESTED LEGISLATION.

(Title, enacting clause, etc.)

Section 1. [This Act may be cited as the *Medically Vulnerable Adults Protection Act*.

Section 2. [*Purpose*.] The Legislature declares that the public policy of this state is to protect adults who, because of physical or mental disability or dependency on institutional services, are particularly vulnerable to abuse or neglect; to provide safe institutional or residential services or living environments for vulnerable adults who have been abused or neglected; and to assist persons charged with the care of vulnerable adults to provide safe environments.

In addition, it is the policy of this state to require reporting of suspected abuse or neglect of vulnerable adults, to provide for the voluntary reporting of abuse or neglect of a medically vulnerable adult, to require the investigation of the reports and to provide protective and counselling services in appropriate cases.

Section 3. [*Definitions*.]

(A) "Abuse" means:
1. Any act which constitutes a violation under [appropriate chapter relating to criminal conduct];
2. Nontherapeutic conduct which produces or could be expected to produce pain or injury and is not accidental; or any repeated conduct which produces or could reasonably be expected to produce mental or emotional distress;
3. Any sexual contact between a facility staff person and a resident or client of that facility;
4. The illegal use of a vulnerable adult person's property for another person's profit or advantage, or the breach of a fiduciary relationship through the use of a person or person's property for any person not in the proper and lawful execution of a trust, including but not limited to situations

where a person obtains money, property, or services from a vulnerable adult through the use of undue influence, harassment, duress, deception or fraud.

5. Counselling or aiding and abetting a suicide, or procuring any lethal instrument or substance when the person procuring these knows or has reason to know that a medically vulnerable adult intends to commit suicide.

(B) "Attending physician" means the physician with primary responsibility for the care and treatment of a patient. If there is more than one physician caring for the patient, these physicians, among themselves, shall designate the "attending physician" for purposes of the Act.

(C) "Caretaker" means an individual or facility who has responsibility for the care of a medically vulnerable adult as a result of family relationship, or who has assumed responsibility for all or a portion of the care of a medically vulnerable adult voluntarily, or by contract, or agreement.

(D) "Facility" means a hospital or other entity required to be licensed pursuant to [appropriate chapter relating to hospitals and other medical facilities]; a nursing home required to be licensed to serve adults pursuant to [appropriate chapter relating to nursing homes]; an agency, day care facility, or residential facility required to be licensed to serve adults pursuant to [appropriate chapter]; or home health agency certified for participation in Titles XVIII or XIX of the Social Security Act, or United States Code, title 42, secs. 1395 et seq.

(E) "Licensing agency" means:

1. The [appropriate commissioner of health] for a facility required to be licensed or certified by the [appropriate department of health];

2. Any [appropriate commissioner of health services] for a facility required to be licensed or certified;

3. Any licensing board which regulates persons pursuant to [appropriate chapter relating to administrative procedure]; and

4. Any agency responsible for credentialing human services occupations.

(F) "Life-resuscitating procedure" means any medical procedure or intervention that uses mechanical or other artificial means to sustain, or supplant a vital function of a person terminally ill and serves only to artificially prolong death. "Life-sustaining procedure" does not include the usual care provided to patients, which would include routine care necessary to sustain patient comfort and the usual and typical provision of nutrition which in the medical judgment of the attending physician such person can tolerate, and subject to the provisions of Section 6.

(G) "Necessary food and water" means nutrition and hydration, irrespective of the manner of provision or assistance, sufficient to maintain the patient at the highest levels of mental and physical functioning as determined by his attending physician in accordance with ordinary and accepted standards of medical care, but does not include nutrition and hydration, when, in the judgment of the patient's attending physician and a second physician:

1. The administration of nutrition and hydration will in and of itself cause severe, intractable, unavoidable and long lasting pain.
2. The administration of nutrition and hydration is not medically feasible, in that:
    a) The patient is unable to ingest nutrients or incorporate fluids, or
    b) No technique or procedure is reasonably available to the attending physician for such administration ; or
3. The death of the patient from a terminal illness is unavoidably imminent.

(H) "Neglect" means:

1. Failure by a caretaker to supply the vulnerable adult with necessary food, water, clothing, shelter, health care or supervision;
2. The absence or likelihood of absence of necessary food, water, clothing, shelter, health care, or supervision.
3. The absence or likelihood of absence of necessary financial management to protect a vulnerable adult against abuse. Nothing in this section shall be construed to require a facility to provide financial management or supervise financial management for a medically vulnerable adult except as otherwise required by law.

(I) "Report" means any report received by a local welfare agency, police department, county sheriff, or licensing agency pursuant to this Act.

(J) "Terminally ill" means the incurable condition of a person caused by injury, disease or illness which, regardless of the application of life-sustaining procedures will, within reasonable medical judgment, produce death, and where the application of life-resuscitating procedures serve only to postpone the moment of death of the person.

(K) "Vulnerable adult" means any person any person 18 years of age or older:

    1. Who is a resident or inpatient of a facility;
    2. Who receives services at or from a facility, except a person receiving outpatient services for treatment of chemical dependency or mental illness;
    3. Who, regardless of residence or type of service received, is unable or unlikely to report abuse or neglect without assistance because of impairment of mental or physical function or emotional status.

Section 4. [*Persons Mandate to Report*.]

(A) A professional or his delegate engaged in the care of vulnerable adults, in education, in social services, law-enforcement, or in any of the regulated occupations referenced in Sections 3(E)(3) and 3(E)(4), or an employee of a rehabilitation facility certified by the [appropriate commissioner of vocational rehabilitation], or an employee of or a person providing services in a facility who has knowledge of the abuse or neglect of a vulnerable adult, has reasonable cause to believe that a vulnerable adult has sustained a physical injury which is not reasonably explained by the history of injuries provided by the caretaker or caretakers of the vulnerable adult shall immediately report the information to the local police department, county sheriff, local welfare agency, or appropriate licensing or certifying agency. Medical examiners or coroners shall notify the police department or county sheriff and the local welfare department in instances in which they believe that a vulnerable adult has died as a result of abuse or neglect. The police department or the county sheriff, upon receiving a report, shall immediately notify the local police department or the county sheriff and the appropriate licensing agency or agencies.

(B) A person required to report under the provisions of the Section may voluntarily report as described above. Nothing in this section shall be construed to require the reporting or transmittal of information regarding an incident of abuse or neglect or suspected abuse or neglect or if the incident has been reported or transmitted to the appropriate person or entity.

Section 5. [*Report Not Required.*]

(A) Where federal law specifically prohibits a person from disclosing patient identifying information in connection with a report of suspected abuse or neglect under this Act, that person need not make a required report unless the vulnerable adult, or the vulnerable adult's guardian, conservator, or legal representative, has consented to disclosure in a manner which confirms to federal requirements. Facilities whose patients or residents are covered by such a federal law shall seek consent to the disclosure of suspected abuse or neglect from each patient or resident, or his guardian, conservator, or legal representative, upon his admission to the facility. Persons who are prohibited by federal law from reporting an incident of suspected abuse or neglect shall promptly seek consent to make a report.

(B) Except as provided in Section 3(A)(1), verbal or physical aggression occurring between patients, residents, or clients of a facility, or self-abusive behavior of these persons does not constitute "abuse" for the purposes of Section 4 unless it causes serious harm. The operator of the facility or a designee shall record incidents of aggression and self-abusive behavior in a manner that facilitates periodic review by licensing agencies and county local welfare agencies.

(C) Nothing in this section shall be construed to require a report of abuse, as defined in Section 3(A)(4), solely on the basis of the transfer of money or property by gift or as compensation for services rendered.

Section 6. [*Report.*] A person required to report under Section 4 shall make an oral report immediately by telephone or otherwise, and shall make a written report as soon as possible thereafter to the appropriate police department, the county sheriff, local welfare agency, or appropriate licensing agency. The written report shall be of sufficient content to identify the vulnerable adult, the caretaker, the nature and extent of the suspected abuse or neglect, name and address of the reporter, and any other information that the reporter believes might be helpful in investigated the suspected abuse or neglect. Written reports received by a police department or a county sheriff shall be forwarded immediately to the local welfare agency. The police department or the county sheriff may keep copies of reports received by them. Copies of written reports received by a local welfare department shall be forwarded immediately to the local police department or county sheriff and the appropriate licensing agency or agencies.

Section 7. [*Immunity From Liability*.]

(A) A person making a voluntary or mandated report under Section 4 or participating in an investigation under this Act is immune from any civil or criminal liability that otherwise might result from the person's actions, if the person is acting in good faith.

(B) A person employed by a local welfare agency or a state licensing agency who is conducting or supervising an investigation or enforcing the law in compliance with sections 12, 13, or 14 or any related rule or provision of law is immune from any civil or criminal liability that might otherwise result from the person's actions, if the person is acting in good faith and exercising due care.

Section 8. [*Falsified Reports*.] A person who intentionally makes a false report under the provisions of this Act shall be liable in a civil suit for any actual damages suffered by the person or persons so reported and for any punitive damages set by the court or jury.

Section 9. [*Failure to Report*.]

(A) A person required to report by this Act who intentionally fails to report is guilty of a misdemeanor.

(B) A person required to report by this Act who negligently or intentionally fails to report is liable for damages caused by the failure.

Section 10. [*Evidence Not Privileged*.] No evidence regarding the abuse or neglect of the vulnerable adult shall be excluded in any proceeding arising out of the alleged abuse or neglect on the grounds of lack of competency under [appropriate evidentiary code section.]

Section 11. [*Mandatory Reporting To A Medical Examiner or Coroner.*] A person required to report under Section 4 who has reasonable cause to believe that a vulnerable adult has died as a direct or indirect result of abuse or neglect, shall report that information to the appropriate medical examiner or coroner in addition to the local welfare agency, policy department, or county sheriff or appropriate licensing agency or agencies. The medical examiner or coroner shall complete an investigation as soon as feasible and report the findings to the police department or county sheriff, the local welfare agency, and if applicable, each licensing agency.

Section 12. [*Duties of Local Welfare Agency Upon Receipt of A Report.*]

(A) The local welfare agency shall immediately investigate and offer emergency and continuing protective social services for purposes of preventing further abuse or neglect and for safeguarding and enhancing the welfare of the abused or neglected vulnerable adult. Local welfare agencies may enter facilities and inspect and copy records as part of investigations. In cases of suspected sexual abuse, the local welfare agency shall immediately arrange for and make available to the victim appropriate medical examination and treatment. The investigation shall not be limited to the written records of the facility, but shall include every other available source of information. When necessary in order to protect the vulnerable adult from further harm, the local welfare agency shall seek authority to remove the vulnerable adult from the situation in which the neglect or abuse occurred. The local welfare agency shall also investigate to determine whether the conditions which resulted in the reported abuse or neglect place other medically vulnerable adults in jeopardy of being abused or neglected and offer protective social services that are called for by its determination. In performing any of these duties, the local welfare agency shall maintain appropriate records.

(B) If the report indicates, or if the local welfare agency finds that the suspected abuse or neglect occurred at a facility, or while the vulnerable adult was or should have been under the care of or receiving services from a facility, or that the suspected abuse or neglect involved a person licensed by a licensing agency to provide care or services, the local welfare agency shall immediately notify each appropriate licensing agency, and provide each licensing agency with a copy of the report and of its investigative findings.

(C) When necessary in order to protect a vulnerable adult from serious harm, the local agency shall immediately intervene on behalf of that adult to help the family, victim, or other interested persons by seeking any of the following:

>1. A restraining order or a court order for removal of the perpetrator from the residence of the vulnerable adult pursuant to [appropriate rule of civil procedure];
>2. The appointment of a guardian or conservator, or guardianship or conservatorship pursuant to [appropriate chapter relating to guardianship];
>3. Replacement of an abusive or neglectful guardian or conservator, pursuant to [appropriate chapter relating to guardianship]; or
>4. A referral to the prosecuting attorney for possible criminal prosecution of the perpetrator under [appropriate criminal procedure section].

(D) The expenses of legal intervention must be paid by the county in the case of indigent persons, under [appropriate section relating to indigence].

(E) In guardianship and conservatorship proceedings, if a suitable relative or other person is not available to petition for guardianship or conservatorship, a county employee shall present the petition with representation by the county attorney. The county attorney shall contract with or arrange for a suitable person or nonprofit organization to provide ongoing guardianship services. If the county presents evidence to the probate court that it has made a diligent effort and no other suitable person can be found, a county employee may serve as guardian or conservator. The county shall not retaliate against the employee for any action taken on behalf of the ward or conservatee even if the action is adverse to the county's interests. Any person retaliated against in violation of this Section shall have a cause for action against the county and shall be entitled to reasonable attorney fees and costs of the action if the action is upheld by the court.

Section 13. [Notification of Neglect or Abuse in a Faculty].

(A) When a report is received that alleging abuse or neglect of a medically vulnerable adult while in the care of a facility required to be licensed under [appropriate chapter relating to nursing homes], or [relating to day care or residential facilities], the local welfare agency investigating the report shall notify the guardian or conservator of the person of a vulnerable adult under guardianship or conservatorship of the person who is alleged to have been abused or neglected. The local welfare agency shall notify the person who is alleged to have been abused or neglected, unless consent is denied by the medically vulnerable adult. The notice shall contain the following information: The name of the facility; the fact that a report of alleged abuse or neglect of a vulnerable adult in the facility has been received, the nature of the alleged abuse or neglect; that the agency is conducting an investigation; any protective or corrective measures being taken pending the outcome of the investigation; and that a written memorandum will be provided when the investigation is completed.

(B) In a case of alleged abuse or neglect of a vulnerable adult while in the care of a facility required to be licensed under [appropriate section relating to day care or residential facilities], the local welfare agency may also provide the information in paragraph (A) or (B): The name of the facility investigated; the nature of the alleged neglect or abuse; the investigator's name' a summary of the investigative findings; a statement of whether the report was found to be substantiated, inconclusive, or false; and the protective or corrective measures that are being or will be taken. The memorandum shall protect the identity of the reporter and the alleged victim and shall not contain the name or, to the extent possible, reveal the identity of the alleged perpetrator or of those interviewed during the investigation.

(C) In a case neglect or abuse of a medically vulnerable adult while in the care of a facility required to be licensed under [appropriate sections relating to day care or residential facilities], the local welfare agency may also provide the written memorandum to the guardian or conservator of the person of any other vulnerable adult in the facility who is under guardianship who is under guardianship or conservatorship of the person, to any other vulnerable adult in the facility who is not under guardianship or conservatorship of the person, and to the person, if any designated to be notified in case of an emergency by any other vulnerable adult in the facility who is not under guardianship or conservatorship of the person, unless consent is denied by the vulnerable adult, if the report is unsubstantiated or if the investigation is inconclusive and the report is a second or subsequent report of neglect or abuse of a medically vulnerable adult while in the care of the facility.

(D) In determining whether to exercise the discretionary authority granted under paragraphs (B) and (D), the local welfare agency shall consider the seriousness and extent of the alleged abuse or neglect and the impact of notification on the residents of the facility. The facility shall be notified whenever this discretion is exercised.

(E) Where federal law specifically prohibits the disclosure of patient identifying information, the local welfare agency shall not provide any notice under paragraph (A) or (B) or any memorandum under paragraph (C) or (D) unless the medically vulnerable adult has consented to disclosure in a manner which conforms to federal requirements.

Section 14. [Duties of Licensing Agencies Upon Receipt of a Report.] Whenever a licensing agency receives a report, or otherwise has information indicating that a vulnerable adult may have been abused or neglected at a facility it has licensed, or that a person it has licensed or credentialed to provide health care or services may be involved in the abuse or neglect of a medically vulnerable adult, or that such a facility or person has failed to comply with the requirements of this Act, it shall immediately investigate. Subject to the [appropriate administrative procedure sections], the licensing agency shall have the right to enter facilities and inspect and copy records as part of investigations. The investigation shall not be limited to the written records of the facility, but shall include every other available source of information. The licensing agency shall issue orders and take actions with respect to the license of the facility or the person that are designated to prevent further abuse or neglect of vulnerable adults.

Section 15. [*Records.*]

(A) Each licensing agency shall maintain summary records of reports of alleged abuse or neglect and alleged violations of the requirements of this section with respect to facilities or persons licensed or credentialed by the agency. As part of these records, the agency shall prepare an investigation memorandum. The investigation memorandum shall be a public record and a copy shall be provided to any public agency which referred the matter to the licensing agency for investigation. It shall contain a complete review of the agency's investigation, including, but not limited to: the name of any facility investigated; a statement of the nature of the alleged abuse or neglect or other violation of the requirements of this section; [pertinent information obtained from medical or other records reviewed; the investigator's name; a summary of the investigation's findings; a statement of whether the report was found to be substantiated, inconclusive or false; and a statement of any action taken by the agency. The investigation memorandum shall protect the identity of the reporter and of the medically vulnerable adult and my not contain the name or, to the extent possible, the identity of the alleged perpetrator or of those interviewed during the investigation. During the licensing agency's investigation, all data collected pursuant to this Act shall be classified as investigative data pursuant to [appropriate administrative code section]. After the licensing agency's investigation is complete, the data on individuals collected and maintained shall be private data on individuals. All data collected pursuant to this section shall be made available to prosecuting authorities and law enforcement officials, local welfare agencies, and licensing agencies investigating the alleged abuse or neglect. Notwithstanding any law to the contrary, the name of the reporter shall be disclosed only upon a finding by the court that the report was false and made in bad faith.

(B) Notwithstanding any law to the contrary,

    1. All data maintained by licensing agencies, treatment facilities, or other public agencies which relate to reports which, upon investigation, are found to be false may be destroyed two years after the finding was made;

    2. All data maintained by licensing agencies, treatment facilities, or other public agencies which relate to reports which, upon investigation, are found to be inconclusive may be destroyed four years after the findings were made;

    3. All data maintained by licensing agencies, treatment facilities, or other public agencies which relate to reports which, upon investigation, are found to be substantiated may

be destroyed seven years after the finding was made.

Section 16. [*Coordination.*]

(A) Any police department or county sheriff, upon receiving a report shall notify the local welfare agency pursuant to Section 4. A local welfare agency or licensing agency which receives a report pursuant to that Section shall immediately notify the appropriate law enforcement, local welfare, and licensing agencies.

(B) Investigating agencies, including the police department, county sheriff, local welfare agency, or appropriate licensing agency shall cooperate in coordinating their investigatory activities. Each licensing agency which regulates facilities shall develop and disseminate procedures to coordinate its activities with:

1. Investigations by police and county sheriffs, and
2. Provision of protective services by local welfare agencies.

Section 17. [*Abuse Prevention Plans.*]

(A) Each facility, except home health agencies, shall establish and enforce an ongoing written abuse prevention plan. The plan shall contain an assessment of the physical plant, its environment, and its population identifying factors which may encourage or permit abuse, and a statement of specific measures to be taken to minimize the risk of abuse. The plan shall comply with any rules governing the plan promulgated by the licensing agency.

(B) Each facility shall develop an individual abuse prevention plan for each vulnerable adult residing or receiving services there. The plan shall contain an individualized assessment of the person's susceptibility to abuse, and a statement of the specific measures to be taken to minimize the risk of abuse to that person. For the purposes of this clause, the term "abuse" includes self-abuse.

Section 18. [*Internal Reporting of Abuse and Neglect.*] Each facility shall establish and enforce ongoing an written procedure in compliance with the licensing agency's rules for insuring that all cases of suspected abuse or neglect are reported and investigated promptly.

Section 19. [*Enforcement.*]

(A) A facility that has not complied with this section within 60 days of the effective date of passage of temporary rules is ineligible for renewal of its license. A person required by Section 4 to report and who is licensed or credentialed to practice the occupation by a licensing agency who willfully fails to comply with this Act shall be disciplined after a hearing by the appropriate licensing agency.

(B) Licensing agencies shall as soon as possible promulgate rules necessary to implement the requirements of sections 14, 15, 16, 17, 18, and 19(A). Agencies may promulgate temporary rules pursuant to [appropriate administrative procedure section].

(C) The [appropriate commissioner of human services] shall promulgate rules as necessary to implement the requirements of section 12.

Section 20. [*Retaliation Prohibited.*]

(A) A facility or person shall not retaliate against any person who reports in good faith suspected abuse or neglect pursuant to this Act, or against a vulnerable adult with respect to whom a report is made, because of the report.

(B) Any facility or person which retaliates against any person because of a report of suspected abuse or neglect is liable to is at person for actual damages and, in addition, a penalty up to $1000.

(C) There shall be a rebuttable presumption that any adverse action, as defined below, within 90 days of a report, is retaliatory. For purposes of this clause, the term "adverse action" refers to action taken by a facility or person involved in a report against the person making the report or the person with respect to whom the report was made because of the report, and includes, but is not limited to:

1. Discharge or transfer from the facility;
2. Discharge or termination of employment;
3. Demotion or reduction in remuneration for services;
4. Restriction or prohibition of access to the facility or its residents; or
5. Any restriction of rights set forth in [appropriate section enumerating employee rights.]

Section 21. [*Outreach.*] the [appropriate commissioner of human services] shall establish an aggressive program to educate those required to report, as well as the general public, about the requirements of this Act using a variety of media.

Section 22. [*Penalty.*] Any caretaker or operator or employee thereof, or volunteer worker thereat, who intentionally abuses or neglects a medically vulnerable adult, or being a caretaker, knowingly permits conditions to exist which result in the abuse or neglect of a vulnerable adult, is guilty of a [serious misdemeanor].

# INDEX

Abortion, 31-63.
Admiraal, Pieter, 138, 143
Adler, Mortimer, 9, 14, 15, 35.
Advance Directives, 125-137.
Aggression, fetal, 42-45.
"Aid-in-Dying", 142-149.
Alzheimer's disease, 182-183, and assisted feeding, 115, 159-164, 182-183.
Annas, George, 96.
American Academy of Pediatrics, 67-77.
American Civil Liberties Union, 109-110.
American Medical Association, 149-150.
American Society of Enteral and Parenteral Nutrition, 198.
Animate-sensate individuals, 9-11.
Anscombe, G.E.M., 14, 35.
Aquinas, Thomas, 151-153, 223.
Arluke, Arnold, 118.
Ashley, Benedict, 34, 38, 226, 249-253, 258.
Assisted feeding, 187-194, 256-262, and common good, 153-169.
Atkinson, Gary, 153-169.

Barber, Neil, 86-89, 236, 257.
Barry, Robert, 52, 91, 164, 191, 272.
Bathhurst, Ella, 94-95, 274-278.
Bayer, Edward, 82, 247-248.
Becker, Lawrence, 24.
Beecher, Henry, 204.
Benefits, of medical treatment, 182-187, of care, 168-169, 263-272.
Bernardin, Cardinal Joseph, 174, 180.
Black, Peter, 209, 212.
Bouvia, Elizabeth, 100-102.
Brain Death, 201-234, and cerebral death, 213, and spontaneous integrated organic functioning, 220-226, concepts of, 217-220, criteria of, 201-217.
Brophy, Paul, 102-105.
Burdens maternal, 45-46, 49-51, fetal, useless, 39-42.
Byrne, Paul, 220.

Callahan, Daniel, 253-354.
Capron, Alexander, 211.
Christa Nursing Home, 93.
Claims, to life, 50-55.
Coma, 86-89, 90-91, 103-109, 111-118, 191, 194, 196, and feeding, 261-2, 87.
Compton, Lynn, 101-102.
Conceptual thought, 15, 17, conditions for ascription, 17-19.
Connery, S.J., John, 239-

242.
Conroy, Claire, 89-93, 257.
Cranford, Ronald, 65-71, 77.
Critical organ, 216-217.
Cronin, Daniel, 167-168.
Cushing, M, 96.

Davies, James, 93-99, 277-280.
Death, definition of, 217-220.
DeLugo, Juan, Cardinal, 157-159.
Dementia and withdrawal of care, 89-93, 182-85.
Dickey, Nancy, 117.
Dignity, death with, 137-149.
Di Ianni, Albert, 24.
Dillon, M.E., 202
Direct killing, of unborn, 53-54, 56-58, by withdrawal of care, 77-80, 91, 109-110, 113-114, 118-119, 120.
Doerflinger, Richard, 121-122, 205, 208, 212.
Donceel, Joseph, 234-4.
Donovan, Joseph, 163.
Doudera, Edward, 65.

Ensoulemnt and abortion, 11-14, 20-29, and brain death, 220-226, and euthanasia, 183.
Euthanasia, and physicians, 142-143 and the law, 139-142, 143, morality of, 142-143, feeding, 180-182, in Holland, 145-146.
Extraordinary means, 159-160, and nutrition and hydration, 162-165, 263-271.

Fenigsen, Ricard, 146.
Finnis, John, 41, 54, 231.
Fletcher, Joseph, 182.
Flieschman, Alan, 69-75.
Food and water, "common", 156-157.
Foot, Philipa, 43.
Freedman, Benjamin, 68, 77.
Freedom and Suicide, 143-145.

Geatch, Peter, 15.
Gerber, Rudolf, 12, 13, 19, 224.
Gilbert, Roswell, 139.
Good Samaritan, 49-58, 176.
Goldman, Edward, 92.
Griese, Orville, 272.
Grant, Edward, 78, 86-9, 193.
Grisez, Germain, 19-20, 25, 32, 37, 63, 246-247, food and water, 262-272.
Guidelines, for withdrawing, 71, in Bouvia, 101-103, in Brophy, 104-105, in Conroy, 92-93, Herbert, 86, in Jobes, 112-116, in Rasmussen, 108, in

# INDEX

handicapped infants, 76-84.
Gunning, K. F. 145-146.

Hannan, Archbishop Philip, 174.
Harp, James, 209.
Harrison, Beverly, 31-32.
Hastings Center, 256-157.
Hemlock Society, 121-124.
Hentoff, Nat, 115.
Heir, Mary, 95-97.
Herbert, Clarence, 86-89.
Hohfeldian Rights, 40-44, 50, 52-54.
Horan, Dennis, 78, 86-9, 193.
Hoyt, Jane, 93-99, 112, 277-280.
Humanoid animals, 201.
Humphry, Derek, 137, 275.
Hunger, as medical condition, 189-190, 236, 258.
Hussman, Joseph, 141.

ICRC's, 125-137, moral responsibilities, 75-84, roles, 67-71.
Identification of persons, demonstrative, 7-8, identifiability-dependence, 7, locatable-sequential-identification, 2-3.
Image of God, 34-39.
Incompetent patients and decision making, 77-81, 271-302, and advance directives, 77-81.
Indirect killing, of unborn, 53-54, 56-58.
Individuality of unborn human life, 19-20.

Janis, I.T, 74.
Jay, Allen, 136.
Jeffcoate, T.N.A., 47.
Jobes, Nancy Ellen, 110-117.
Johnstone, Brian, 272.
Jonas, Hans, 215, 219.

Kass, Leon, 273.
Kew Gardens principle, 75.
Kelly, Gerald, 159-167, 238-239, 242.
Klubertantz, George, 223.
Koop, C. Everett, 113-114.
Korein, Julius, 207, 219.
Kushner, T, 74.

Lamb, David, 206, 210, 216.
LaRue, G, 164.
Law, Cardinal Bernard, 174, 181.
Law, and assisted feeding, 262-271, and euthanasia, 273-302, and suicide,139-142 and the federal government, 281-284, and the states, 284-285.
Lebowitz, Lawrence, 105.
Lethal injections, 143, 137.
Levin, Jack, 118.
Levine, Carol, 65, 68-73.
Lifton, Robert, 143.

Lo, Bernard, 72, 73.
Lonergan, Bernard, 32.

Mahony, Archbishop Roger, 174, 181.
Maloney, S.J, George, 35.
Marker, Rita, 119, 127.
Marmorstein, Jerome, 119.
Marzen, Thomas, 121, 125-137, 272.
Material individuals, 2-7.
May, William, E, 31, 75, 186, 244-246, 260, 263-271.
Mayo, David, 121-123, 142-143.
McCartney, James, 11.
McCormick, Richard, 66, 183, 195, 238-239.
McFadden, Charles, 171-172.
McGuire, Daniel, 100.
McHugh, Bishop James, 272.
McHugh, Charles, 77.
Meilander, Gilbert, 114, 272.
  human states of mind, 13.
Miles, Stephen, 189-190.
Minimal Care, 254-256.
Modes of Identification of material individuals, 7-9.
Nasogastric tubes and catheters, 88-89, 91, 257-260, and respirators, 257-8.
National Conference of Catholic Bishops, 179-180, 229.
National Conference of Commissioners of Uniform State Laws, 125-137.
Nejdl, Robert, 86-89.
Non-transferable character of states of mind, 16-17.
Neomorts, 205-6.
New Jersey Catholic Conference, 112, 181.
New Jersey Supreme Court, 91- 93, 111-116.
NINCDS Collaborative Study on Brain Death, 210, 227.
Non-public observability of states of mind, 16.

O'Connor, Cardinal, John, 181.
O'Connell, Laurence, 149-150.
O'Donnell, Thomas, 230, 160, 242-244.
Ordinary means, 133, and "useless" means, 242-244, normal care, 190n, 258-262, food and water, 20-29, and feeding, 194.
Organ Transplants, and brain death, 205-207.
O'Rourke, Kevin, 35, 38, 179-199, 226, 258.

Pallis, James, 206.
Paris, John, 236-238, 257, 258.
Quality of life, 180n, 183
Quay, Paul, 220.

Ramsey, Paul, 31, 159.

## INDEX

Rango, Nicholas, 120.
Rape and abortion, 46, 50-53.
Rasmussen, Mildred, 107-109.
Requenna, Beverly, 105-107.
Repsonsive capabilities of animate individuals, 10.
Retention of particulars of material individuals, 5-6.
Right to life, 58-63.
Rights, of unborn child and of mother, 39-57.
Risley, Robert, 121.
Rizzo, Robert, 225.
Rodas, Hector, 109-110.
Rollin, Betty, 275.

Sacred Congregation for the Doctrine of the Faith, 79, 174, 192, 281.
Schiffer, R. B., 210.
Schwager, Robert, 212.
Shaneyfelt, David, 284.
Shewman, D. Alan, 194, 201-234.
Siebert, Sharon, 93-5.
Siegler, Mark, 203, 205, 208, 272.
Singer, Peter, 27.
Smith, William, 164, 254-256, 259, 272.
Smith, David, 120.
Society for the Right to Die, 125, 275.
Spatio-temporal identifiability, 3-5.
Stanley, Lisa, 242.
Stein, Robert, 111-113.
Steinbock, Bonnie, 86-88.

Strawson, Peter, 2-18.
Suicide, assisted, morality of, 144.
Sullivan, John, 34, 36-37.
Sullivan, Joseph, 169-171.
Sumners, J. W. 72.
Syntactical, propositional speech and persons, 16-17.

Tangibility of material individuals, 4.
Temporally existing states of mind, 11.
Terminal illness, 129-130.
Therapy and maternal support, 46-47, and assisted feeding, 187-193, 259-261.
Thomson, Judith, Jarvis, 31, 38-63.
Tooley, Michael, 22-29.
Traits, of material animate individuals, 2-7, of persons, 11-19.
Tredgold, R.G. 47.

Uniform Rights of the Terminally Ill Act, 125-137.

Value, of person, 32-39.

Van Till, Adrienne, 208-218, 219.
Veatch, Henry, 210, 213,

Veith, Frank, 211, 213, 217.
Vitoria, Francisco, 153-157.

Waller, Susan, 122.
Walton, Douglas, 205-219, 233.
Weir, Robert, 81-4.
Welty, Eberhard, 165-167.

Werthem, Fredrick, 140.
Wikler, Daniel, 205.
Winslow, G., 72.
Withdrawing, maternal support, 39-49.
Wylie, Philip, 31.
Wynan, Andre, 118.

Yonder, Paul, 225.
Youngner, Stuart, 72.

Anthony J. Blasi

# MORAL CONFLICT AND CHRISTIAN RELIGION

American University Studies: Series VII (Theology and Religion). Vol. 35
ISBN 0-8204-0497-7      190 pages      hardback US $ 33.50*

*Recommended price – alterations reserved

This work takes up the problem of moral conflict, wherein a person must choose between two or more evils. The problem lies behind such issues as the defensive war, therapeutic abortion, and contraception. It becomes a religious question because, as the author argues, religion elicits the same kind of openness to values as is needed for addressing moral dilemmas. After culling insights out of the history of Christian ethics, Blasi presents phenomenologies of both moral decision making and religion, and uses the results to address the variety of moral dilemmas.

«This is an original and enlightening study of a timely and important subject.» (Leslie Dewart, St. Michael's College, University of Toronto)

«Conflict situations will always exist. And therefore so will the need for thoughtful precision in dealing with them. Blasi's book is a significant contribution to that precision.» (Richard A. McCormick, S. J., University of Notre Dame)

«... the work represents a very original and inspiring contribution to moral inquiry ...» (Béla Somfai, Regis College).

PETER LANG PUBLISHING, INC.
62 West 45th Street
USA – New York, NY 10036

James J. McCartney

# UNBORN PERSONS
Pope John Paul II and the Abortion Debate

American University Studies: Series VII (Theology and Religion). Vol. 21
ISBN 0-8204-0349-0          176 pages          hardback US $ 28.95*

*Recommended price – alterations reserved

Karol Wojtyla (Pope John Paul II) was a professor of anthropology and ethics at the Catholic University of Lublin, Poland long before he was elected Pope. During this time, his interests centered around the concept of personhood and its many implications in the epistemological, metaphysical and ethical spheres. In this book, after considering the many philosophical and theological influences that helped to form his tought, his notion of personhood is discussed with reference to the status of unborn persons, that is of embryological and fetal life. His approach to personhood is then contrasted and compared with other contemporary notions in an effort to understand more clearly the status of life before birth.

Contents: Theological and Philosophical Influences on Wojtyla's Notion of «Person» – A Dialogue between Wojtyla and Others on Whether or Not the Living Human Embryo is a Person.

*«To relate Wojtyla's (Pope John Paul II's) more general philosophical and theological thought to his notion of personhood (its beginning, constitutive elements, etc.) is a valuable piece of research. It is what James J. McCartney has done in this careful and well-crafted study.»*
(Reverend Richard A. McCormick, S. J.)

PETER LANG PUBLISHING, INC.
62 West 45th Street
USA – New York, NY 10036